Nursing Research I

Nursing Research I

Edited by Phyllis J. Verhonick, R.N., Ed.D.
Professor of Nursing and Director of Research
School of Nursing, University of Virginia
Charlottesville

With 10 Contributing Authors

LITTLE, BROWN AND COMPANY, BOSTON

Nursing Research I

First Edition

Library of Congress catalog card No. 74-6604

ISBN 0-316-90010-9

Printed in the United States of America

To Leona Louise Verhonick
for many years of continued support

Contributing Authors

JEANNE QUINT BENOLIEL, R.N., D.N.Sc.
Professor and Chairman, Comparative Nursing Care Systems Department
School of Nursing
University of Washington
Seattle

JAMES DICKOFF, Ph.D.
Professor of Philosophy
Kent State University
Kent, Ohio

SHERRY ISRAEL, Ph.D.
Lecturer, Foundations of Education Department
College of Education
Northeastern University
Boston

PATRICIA JAMES, Ph.D.
Professor of Philosophy
Kent State University
Kent, Ohio

IMOGENE M. KING, R.N., Ed.D.
Professor, School of Nursing
Loyola University
Chicago

ROBERT C. LEONARD, Ph.D.
Professor, Sociology Department
University of Arizona
Tucson

HOWARD LEVENTHAL, Ph.D.
Professor, Department of Psychology
University of Wisconsin
Madison

ROZELLA M. SCHLOTFELDT, R.N., Ph.D., D.Sc.
Professor, Frances Payne Bolton School of Nursing
Case Western Reserve University
Cleveland

JAMES K. SKIPPER, Jr., Ph.D.
Professor of Sociology, Department of Social Medicine
Medical College of Ohio at Toledo
Toledo

POWHATAN J. WOOLDRIDGE, Ph.D.
Professor of Sociology, Departments of Nursing and Sociology
University of Rochester
Rochester, New York

Preface

THIS book is on the subject of research in nursing. It is planned to be a valuable reference, presenting underlying philosophy, research needs, and general background in the areas covered. The research process is described in detail, and examples from actual investigations in the field of nursing are used to illustrate approaches and techniques.

The authors who have been invited to contribute to the series, of which this is the first volume, all have wide experience and a deep interest in nursing research – whether as practitioner-investigators, researchers in related scientific areas, or theorists. Many of the nurses who are contributors also have preparation in other disciplines; basically they are all striving to bridge the gap between nursing and other areas of scientific endeavor.

Nurses will reach professional status through research, coupled with excellence in education and expertise in practice. The evolution over the two decades since nursing research came alive in 1950 has shown that there are many approaches to the study of nursing. This book will present the approaches that have been most fruitful.

The focus is on general methodology rather than on detailed methodological steps. Thus the content will encompass the concepts and theories basic to nursing, physiological and biological research methods, behavioral science research approaches, clinical investigations, and systems and operations research concerned with nursing and health care. Guidelines for problems encountered in the conduct of research will be provided, rather than detailed steps in methodology.

The material is designed to meet the needs of the beginning researcher. Those who have received a master's or doctoral degree and plan a career of continued research will find that the general approaches and orientation toward specific problems will serve as guidelines for carrying out their own investigations. It is this philosophy that will permeate the series.

P. J. V.

Charlottesville

Contents

The Conceptual Framework of Nursing Research

I

THE development of a conceptual or theoretical framework is the fundamental process required before conducting actual research. This elementary step has frequently been difficult for nurses to understand. Research in nursing is relatively new, and the discipline of conceptualizing and identifying its theoretical bases is an unfamiliar exercise to many beginning investigators. In the practice of nursing we are not, generally, accustomed to the process of thinking conceptually.

The three chapters of Part I provide general information on the importance of concept and theory formation, with examples that relate to nursing and patient care. There is a great need to provide a foundation of nursing knowledge as we struggle to identify ourselves as a true profession. The concepts and theories developed and then verified through nursing research will help to build a sound scientific approach. The scholarly endeavors of critical thinking, extensive literature review, and the search for logical relationships between the abstract and reality are outlined throughout this part.

Dr. Schlotfeldt emphasizes the need for conceptual frameworks for nursing investigation. This is the beginning step for any systematic investigation. The study of nursing is not examined in a vacuum; investigations in parent disciplines are also discussed. Specific examples related to patient care help to illustrate the manner in which conceptualization works. The importance of conceptualization in nursing is expressed in terms of needed knowledge for the attainment of goals and guides for investigation.

In Chapter 2, Dr. King considers the relevance of concept development in nursing. Models illustrate the relationship between nursing practice, research, and concept formation. The process of concept development for nursing is briefly covered in terms of inductive and deductive approaches. A specific theoretical framework with four major concepts is outlined to serve as a guide for nurse-investigators.

Research in a service discipline is difficult, but specific nursing acts inherent in the art of the practice have a bearing on the development of a nursing theory. The relationship of theory, research, and practice is important for both researchers and practitioners of nursing. The final chapter in Part I by Doctors Dickoff and James deals with the development of theory generally and as applied to nursing. These two philosophers provide guidelines for theory formation and discuss four levels of theory basic to nursing research.

The Need for a Conceptual Framework

Rozella M. Schlotfeldt

I

SYSTEMATIC inquiry, whether it is carried out for the purpose of resolving commonsense problems, verifying trends, determining the status of circumstances or events, establishing the existence of order in a set of observations, or identifying causal relationships or antecedents to consequences, requires a conceptual guide or intellectual focus for the inquirer's observations – if the findings from such inquiry are to be meaningful. Such a guide or focus is a conceptual framework.

The purpose of this chapter is to illustrate how different conceptual schemes influence the nature of the inquiry undertaken, the methods of study utilized, and the findings that derive therefrom. The chapter further addresses the question of approaches to identifying conceptual schemes for the organization of the knowledge of practice disciplines. Several basic assumptions are made explicit.

BASIC ASSUMPTIONS

Research is pursued for the ultimate purpose of advancing knowledge (science). Systematic inquiry is a means to that end. The

Partially supported by Research Development Grant 5 RO2 NU 000 69, Division of Nursing, United States Public Health Service, Department of Health, Education, and Welfare.

research process itself proceeds in a reasonably orderly way from identifying (conceptualizing) a research problem; to gathering, ordering, reducing, and analyzing data; and then to interpreting the findings in relation to the hypotheses, questions, or purposes guiding the investigation. This chapter is concerned with the conceptualizing phase of the research endeavor.

The second assumption basic to the discussion to follow is that there is a body of knowledge unique to each practice discipline and that such a body of knowledge must be continuously advanced and restructured through research. Such a body of knowledge, when mastered by practitioners, is that which makes their efforts scientific, intellectual, and effective. Nursing, like all other practice professions, is an intellectual discipline whose scope of practice requires a constantly changing and expanding body of knowledge, verified through research.

The third assumption basic to this discussion is that science can be communicated because it is embodied in sentences and transmitted through verbal and written discourse. Excluded from this interpretation of science is intuitive knowledge and that which is transmitted solely through example. Because such "knowledge" cannot be subjected to intellectual scrutiny and because nothing can be said about it, it cannot be transmitted and cannot be verified through systematic inquiry. Knowledge as conceived in this discussion is that developed through the orderly process of research, that which is formulated in linguistic symbols, and that which can be acquired only through reading and discourse.

A fourth assumption closely related to the foregoing is that there is a difference between command of knowledge of a practice discipline (verified through research) and possession of knowledge that derives merely from carrying out activities associated with that profession in a practice setting. Nursing science, transmissible through linguistic symbols, is essential to the professional's performance. Of course, competence in practice is equally as important to the professional as knowing about the practice discipline and possessing knowledge of it. The point here made is that even though persons other than professionals can and do carry out some nursing activities, one cannot be a competent, effective, professional practitioner without mastering knowledge of the discipline. Knowledge of the field as conceived here is that which has been confirmed as valid, or at least as highly probable. It is employed selectively, artfully, and skillfully by professionals in the resolution of problems unique to the practice of nursing.

A fifth assumption is that theorists and investigators attempting to structure a science must be knowledgeable about the practice discipline in question and the focus, scope, and limitations of its concerns and responsibilities. In order to investigate nursing questions, the inquirer must be able to identify nursing questions and to pursue the search for knowledge relevant thereto. This assumption does not imply that scientists in other disciplines cannot make contributions to nursing science, or that certain concepts of nursing science may not have relevance for some of the "basic" disciplines and for other professional practice fields as well.

A sixth assumption is that science is now and will continue to be under development. To date, the research endeavor in nursing has been relatively modest. However, the number of scientist nurses is increasing, and they are involving themselves more and more in research that is providing the knowledge base for practice. Nurse-scholars are also engaged in theorizing and subjecting theoretical formulations to rigorous tests with a view toward structuring a body of verified nursing science. Their conceptualizations of the questions and problems of significance to nursing and of the phenomena to be studied have affected, and will continue to affect, the nature of nursing science.

The foregoing discussion has made explicit the expectation that the research endeavor should contribute to the advancement and continuous restructuring of a body of knowledge unique to a practice discipline and capable of being transmitted. Implied in that discussion is the expectation that educational institutions will continue to prepare competent practitioners by providing students with learning opportunities enabling them to master essential intellectual constructs and practitioner skills and, in addition, to develop interests, habits, and attitudes that will motivate them effectively toward continuous learning and efficient performance throughout their careers as practitioners.

Educators in professional practice disciplines have a second obligation. Not only are they expected to keep their knowledge and skills current as practitioners, but they are also required to be competent educators. Nurse-educators are therefore expected to be knowledgeable and proficient in two practice disciplines: nursing and education. The science of education can be considered to be comparable to the science of nursing in that it is unique to the practice discipline, capable of being communicated, and highly tentative.

The need for extensive research in the fields of nursing and education is clearly evident when evaluations are made about the existing bodies of knowledge unique to each of these disciplines. At best, much of the knowledge used as bases for both nursing and educational practices can be looked on as sets of commonsense observations, testimonials concerning traditionally effective practices, prescriptions made without facts to substantiate their value, or unconfirmed hypotheses and imprecise theoretical formulations. In order to have well-confirmed statements that can qualify as components of bodies of valid science basic to the practice fields of nursing and education, both need competent investigators and able theorists whose work will continuously advance and restructure knowledge.

Practice disciplines such as dentistry, education, engineering, medicine, and nursing utilize intellectual constructs from several fields of human knowledge, as well as those unique to each profession. Several conceptual schemes are therefore likely to be employed in organizing and structuring a body of knowledge that will qualify as being unique to each profession. Those same approaches are equally useful in selecting conceptual frameworks for research endeavors undertaken to advance knowledge of the practice fields in question.

CONCEPTUAL APPROACHES TO ADVANCING AND STRUCTURING KNOWLEDGE

Several general approaches have been used to study questions or problems assumed to be of importance to nursing. The reader should recognize that those selected are illustrative only and are not exhaustive. It should also be noted that conceptualization of a research problem must partly reveal the investigator's conceptualization of the discipline under study – if indeed the investigator expects to have research findings contribute to advancing its knowledge base. The conceptual framework selected for a research problem influences (1) the precise nature of the problem to be studied, or the purposes to be fulfilled by the investigation, or both; (2) the phenomena to be studied; (3) the research techniques to be employed and the research tools to be used; (4) the settings in which data are to be gathered and the subjects who are to provide the data; (5) the methods to be employed in reducing and analyzing the data; and (6) the nature of contributions that the research will make to the advancement of knowledge.

CONCEPTUALIZING NURSING QUESTIONS WITHIN BASIC SCIENCE FRAMEWORKS

One approach to conceptualizing nursing's research questions is within a framework of a basic or parent discipline. This approach has persisted over the years and will undoubtedly continue to be utilized by investigators, whether the investigators are scientist nurses or other scientists contributing to the advancement of nursing science or of other fields of knowledge useful to nurses. The tardiness of nursing to develop its own investigators has encouraged researchers other than nurses to conceptualize research problems that are of interest to nurses within frameworks appropriate to their own fields of specialization. Some nurse investigators also study problems exclusively by using concepts borrowed from basic disciplines. It is, of course, logical and appropriate for some investigators to conceptualize man in terms of his physiological, psychological, or social behavior, or his cultural mores and to study his behavior within such frameworks.

Although a parent body of knowledge provides a structure for conceptualizing and studying questions of importance to nurses within a framework appropriate for that discipline, there are some obvious shortcomings to this approach. The first of these relates to the tentative state of all knowledge and to deficiencies in any parent science at any point in time. The tendency of nurse investigators to rely on behavioral science concepts as appropriate guides for their observations in the study of nursing questions is particularly relevant to this point. The behavioral sciences are among the newer disciplines, and many of their concepts and theoretical constructs are as yet unverified [2]. It should be noted that although the natural sciences are much more adequately structured than are the behavioral sciences, they, too, continuously undergo change. Confusion and errors that exist in a parent discipline will, of course, be reflected in the conceptualizations that are selected as appropriate for the study of nursing questions and in findings that derive therefrom. Further, when a problem that is of concern to nurses is formulated in terms of a relevant basic discipline, the inquiry will usually be constricted within a conceptual or theoretical framework that is narrowly focused. Third, findings that derive from an inquiry formulated as an investigation in a basic science can be expected to advance that field of human knowledge, but cannot be expected *as a first priority* to advance knowledge of the practice discipline of nursing. Some illustrations will suffice to point up conceptualizations of problems that are of significance to the profession of nursing within the context of basic or parent disciplines.

Conceptualizations of Pain

The phenomenon of pain is one that nurses experience daily in their work. The advancement of knowledge about pain (in the sense of knowledge as previously described) can be conceived to be an appropriate research objective for scientists of several kinds: biological scientists, behavioral scientists, cultural scientists, and nursing scientists, among others. The nature of pain as a neurophysiological phenomenon was studied extensively by one group of investigators who drew conclusions about the physiological aspects of pain [7]. Such knowledge is useful to nurses as well as to other practitioners in the health care system. Hardy and his associates pointed up differences between conceptualizing pain as a physiological phenomenon and as an "experience of pain," which is endured or accepted in varying ways by persons having the experience [8]. Conceptualizing pain as a human experience undoubtedly stimulated other investigators to study reactions to pain as they are exemplified by individuals representative of particular groups.

One investigator (a social scientist) was led to study attitudes toward and reactions to pain characteristically manifested by members of different ethnocultural groups [24]. Zborowski's stated purpose was not only to contribute to theory related to the pain experience, but also to make a contribution to nursing and medical practices. Through interviews, he obtained statements about the pain experience and reactions to it as reported by Jews, Italians, Irish, and "old Americans" who were suffering from neurological diseases. The investigator's purpose was to be able to make generalizations about reactions to pain as they were exemplified by subjects representing the four ethnocultural groups under study. Although individual differences were noted and reported, and other variables such as sex, age, and the educational backgrounds of subjects were recognized as influencing their reactions, the investigator fulfilled his research objective by establishing culture as a significant determinant of human beings' reactions to the pain experiences.

The conceptual framework guiding this research was one which led a social scientist to design and carry out an inquiry so that he could make valid generalizations about culture as a variable related to peoples' reactions to pain. Knowledge of the attitudes and mores of various representatives of the cultural groups under study was advanced by this investigation; and as a concomitant, information useful to nurses and other practitioners in the field of health care was made available. Judicious use of such knowledge in practice certainly can alert practitioners to cultural factors that might have an influence on an individual patient's reactions to pain. Uncritical acceptance by practicing nurses of generalizations of cultural determinants of patients' reaction to pain, however, could lead them to unwarranted and biased conclusions when interpreting clinical data manifested by an individual member of a cultural group. The point here made is that it is the responsibility of nurses to incorporate knowledge such as that cited above into organized nursing science in such a way as to make its application appropriate and useful.

Conceptualizing pain as a neurological phenomenon or the experience of pain as a phenomenon to which persons react in ways influenced by their cultural backgrounds is inappropriate for the nurse investigator who wishes to study pain as a nursing problem and by so doing, as a first priority, contribute to the advancement of nursing knowledge. This statement does not deprecate the importance of the studies cited; instead, it points up the need for nurse investigators to study the phenomenon within conceptual frameworks that are uniquely relevant to pain as a problem with which patients must cope and nurse practitioners must deal knowledgeably. Findings from systematic inquiry conducted within such frameworks will contribute to the body of nursing science.

Conceptualizations of Death

The phenomenon of death is one which holds great significance for nurses and one which is now being studied in several contexts. The work of Glaser and Strauss [5] illustrates conceptualization of the dying process within a social science framework.

Glaser and his associates inquired into interactional situations surrounding dying patients. The investigators' explicit goal was to develop substantive social theory that could have practical application in the management of the dying process. These investigators pointed up that the "awareness" theory, which they formulated as a result of their research, holds promise of contributing to the development of more general, formal, sociological theory by providing a paradigm for study of a wide variety of interactions.

Glaser and Strauss focused their observations on events occurring between and among persons in a well-defined social system – hospitals in which patients and staff interacted while the dying process was exemplified. They collected only data relevant to the concept of awareness, as revealed in situations in which death was anticipated and those in which death occurred. All other events surrounding the dying process were excluded from their observations. Such exclusion was entirely appropriate for social scientists whose mission was the development of social theory. Glaser and Strauss' substantive findings and their presenting the "awareness" theory certainly are of interest to and useful for practicing nurses. This theoretical construct should be properly incorporated into the body of knowledge known as nursing science. Nursing problems attendant to death also merit investigation. Such inquiries, however, should not be limited to problems cast in the social interactional situation framework, or to studies designed within the context of awareness.

Nurses' responsibilities relevant to the phenomenon of death include their being helpful to persons for whom death is imminent, unanticipated, and predicted to occur within definitive time periods. They also include acting to help and sustain survivors during the immediate circumstances of death and in some situations, over time. The nature and scope of nursing practice and the knowledge nurses need about death and the dying process point up the importance of nurse investigators' identifying conceptual frameworks that require observations uniquely relevant to nurses, and for their designing research that holds promise of contributing to the advancement and structure of nursing knowledge.

CONCEPTUALIZING NURSING AS TASKS

In contrast to investigating nursing questions and problems in terms of conceptual frameworks borrowed from the several parent fields of the natural, social, and behavioral sciences, some investigators have conceptualized nursing as a set of tasks or activities. Thus they conceive nursing practice in terms of categories of functions: (1) performing specific tasks or procedures, (2) counseling, (3) teaching, (4) administering, and (5) executing therapies according to doctors' orders. Conceptualizing nursing as a set of discrete tasks leads to inquiry into the major activities in which nurses consistently and characteristically engage. Such research usually seeks to provide knowledge that will illuminate and, if applied in practice, make more proficient the execution of nurses' tasks. Task analyses are also useful in recording practices in effect at any particular time.

There are obvious limitations to conceptualizing nursing, or any other professional practice discipline, as a set of discrete tasks to be accomplished. The first of these is the assumption of constancy in what practitioners do. With advancements in knowledge and technology and by agreement among practitioners, those with whom they work, and those they serve, practices change remarkably over time. Indeed, some tasks or activities become obsolete as concepts of health care change and as new knowledge, techniques, therapies, devices, instruments, and services become available for practitioners' use. Second, research that conceptualizes professional practice as a set of tasks makes either assumptions or inferences about the knowledge base needed for their accomplishment. Third, research based on task analysis has inherent limitations with regard to the generation of new knowledge in that the main goal is efficiency and effectiveness of observable performance, rather than the generation of theoretical or scientific constructs that are essential, cognitive guides for professional practice.

Task Analyses Studies

Readers acquainted with the history of nursing will recall that two of the earliest studies of nursing reported in the United States had as their object of study identification of the activities in which nurses then engaged. In 1918, the Committee for the Study of Nursing Education employed investigators who observed public health nurses at work and recorded their activities as performed in several settings [3]. In 1934, Johns and Pfefferkorn [11] reported findings from an activity analysis of nursing that was part of a larger inquiry concerned not only with what nurses were then doing, but also with supply and demand factors and conditions existing in schools of nursing in the third decade of this century. It is not surprising that recommendations for learning opportunities to be provided nursing students were inferred directly from information gleaned from activities in which nurses were then engaged. Regrettably, preparation for doing rather than knowing has continued to characterize many nursing school curricula until recently, when educators have begun to place high value on conceptualizing nursing as an intellectual practice discipline. The knowledge base for nursing practice is continuously advanced by research; but conceptualizing nursing as a set of tasks will not generate research that adds significantly to that knowledge base.

In 1966, Kenneth Barker [1], a pharmacologist, reported findings from a study of the incidence of medication errors in a hospital. In his conceptualization of nursing and of his research question, the practitioner who played the nurse role without error was obliged to follow rigidly the doctor's written order for administering medicaments. Barker's method of study was direct observation of nurses executing the task of administering drug therapies to hospitalized patients. His criteria for determining errors included all omission and "delays" in giving medicaments to patients, giving them incorrect drugs and inaccurate amounts of drugs, and administration without a written order. His findings and conclusions related ostensibly to the need for more efficient task performance.

Judgments concerning the efficacy of nursing practice as it relates to administration of medicaments, however, requires inquiry not only into task performance but also into factors that lead nurses to delay or withhold medicaments when contraindications exist and those that prompt them to give medicine without an order when circumstances dictate that by so doing patients are well served. Research designed within a conceptual framework that permits, and indeed requires, inquiry into the intellectual processes that lead to nurses' decisions about therapies is the only approach that holds promise for advancing the knowledge base of nursing practice. In contrast, findings from task analyses hold little promise of improving practice, except as they reveal incompetencies and inappropriate use of practitioners' time. Conclusions concerning inappropriateness of tasks of course require some consensus about the activities in which professionals should engage.

Studies of nurses' and physicians' activities have captured the interest of those who are eager to engage in critical analyses of the costs of patient services or to have the talents of practitioners fully utilized. Findings from studies recently reported do indeed point up the need for decisions concerning the nature of nursing and medical practices, the relationships that should exist between practitioners of both professions, and the expectations that should be held for each type of practitioner [13, 23]. Inquiries into both nursing and medical practices designed to advance knowledge of each practice discipline, however, require that each investigator conceptualize professional practice in relation to its intellectual concerns, rather than as a set of tasks to be performed.

THE SYSTEMS APPROACH TO CONCEPTUALIZING NURSING QUESTIONS

The systems approach to the study of a wide variety of social problems and human endeavors is gaining in popularity. It is broadly described as a means through which to make decision-making scientific and effective [4]. Although it has been recognized by some investigators as a useful approach for nursing, little research utilizing a systems or operations approach has to date been reported in the nursing literature. Its increasing popularity as a tool of management, government, and industry and as an approach to conceptualizing the problems of society in general would lead to the expectation that nursing problems will increasingly be investigated within several "systems" conceptual models.

The allure of the systems approach lies in the intent of its advocates to allocate resources and to utilize existing knowledge to attain objectives that are deemed to be of value for all, while at the same time to avoid disadvantage to any one group. Notions of efficiency, scientific management, information processing, model building, cost benefits, and rational planning are basic to the several conceptual schemes utilized by operations or systems researchers.

Problems Conceptualized in Systems Approach

A systems approach to study of the utilization of health care personnel was reported by Hallstrom [6]. The conceptual model used assumed a flow of clients to be served through a system of care provided by a mix of actors whose functions were described as "independent," "dependent," and "collaborative," as determined by their knowledge and competence. A test was made of the "theoretical" notion that some functions are independent and others delegated or collaborative for particular categories of personnel. The findings demonstrated considerable lack of consensus as to the functions deemed appropriate for particular categories of personnel as revealed in current practices. Hallstrom's conclusion pointed up the need for a larger data base. She anticipated additional studies that would seek data about the availability of various categories of workers and salaries. Notions of efficiency and rational planning to achieve maximum cost benefits through optimal utilization of personnel are implicit in those comments.

Newton and her associates [15] reported an investigation of nursing action in relief of pain through a systems approach to processing information. They conceptualized the nurse, patient, and physician as a triad for the generation and processing of information concerning patients' pain experiences. The investigators designed three models of the information processing system. The first was in terms of its components, the nurse-patient-physician triad. The second model was one in which the components were defined more fully in terms of their attributes. The third model demonstrated relationships between the variables manifested by the components. The third model required that the investigators develop a rating scale for use of observers who recorded intensity of and therefore "measured" pain according to six observed variables. Through factor analysis of the data obtained, a method was devised to express with a relatively small degree of error the intensity of patients' pain experiences as observed by nurses.

The investigators carried their research to the point of building a pain simulator that was capable of demonstrating functional relationships between and among the variables associated with the model's components. According to the investigators, the approach developed demonstrated that experimental studies not possible in the nurse-patient setting could be simulated. They concluded that the systems model-building approach holds promise of contributing to the development of nursing theories.

Model building and computer simulation of the real world are important aspects of the systems approach to inquiry. Theoretically, the scientist and the planner can join forces in making wise decisions about important questions if objectives can be delineated and the consequences of their attainment predicted; and if both can be quantified in terms of their relative values.

A nursing investigation designed within the IDEALS systems methodology [14] did in fact test the feasibility of deliberately restructuring a patient care system in terms of purposes to be attained, based on delineation of patients' requirements [16]. Explication of both goals to be attained and of criteria that served as measures of effectiveness made it possible for investigators to design and test four major systems that were identified as important components of patient care.

Inasmuch as the systems scientist relies on accurate input based on verified knowledge from several decision-makers, identification of gaps in information had by nurses serving as decision-makers and revealed through research designed according to systems models can be expected to point up the need for research in nursing which focuses on the knowledge needed to attain agreed-upon goals.

CONCEPTUALIZING NURSING IN TERMS OF THE KNOWLEDGE NEEDED TO ATTAIN GOALS

Another approach to conceptualizing nursing and nursing's research questions is in terms of knowledge needed to attain explicit goals. This conceptual approach requires rationalization of nursing's raison d'être and explicit statements of the specific goals or desired outcomes of nursing practice. Knowledge, as previously defined, becomes the means for attaining those desired ends. Following this schema the gamut of nursing practice must be conceptualized in terms of nursing's central focus and definitive goals. Nursing's research questions must be formulated and data gathered, reduced, and analyzed within such conceptual frameworks. The ultimate research aim is to advance and structure a body of nursing science which, when applied in practice, holds promise of attaining those explicit goals.

Nurse investigators are now heeding the admonition that the nursing profession needs to have a structured body of nursing knowledge that has direct relevance for professional practice. To obtain verified nursing knowledge, the focus of inquiry must be primarily on persons served, rather than on practitioners and their characteristics, on specific sets of tasks in which practitioners engage at any point in time, or on the cost benefits deriving therefrom. Professionals in nursing need to be concerned primarily with the knowledge base of their practices, namely, its formulation and structure, its transmission through discourse, its application in practice, and its continuous advancement, refinement, and restructuring through scientific inquiry. The raison d'être of nursing provides a conceptual scheme both for structuring nursing science and for conceptualizing specific research problems.

Nursing practice can be conceptualized broadly to be application of knowledge (science) and utilization of a variety of strategies with the goal of stimulating man's health-seeking behavior. This includes enhancing his motivation to attain and retain maximum health and function, to avoid disease and disability, and to attain or regain the highest possible level of health, function, and productivity when he is afflicted with genetic inadequacy, injury, disease, and deprivation of several kinds [20]. Following this schema, the focus of nursing research designed to advance nursing science is on man's health-seeking behaviors – physiological, psychological, social, voluntary and involuntary, conscious and preconscious or subconscious, individual, and group. Since nursing is health care, health-seeking behaviors of individuals, families, communities, and the gamut of social and cultural groups are the phenomena providing the focus for nursing research that seeks to identify the knowledge (science) base for practice.

The figure presents a schematic conceptualization of man's health-seeking behavior (and nursing practice) in terms of outcomes. At the extreme right of the diagram are goals assumed to be sought by individuals and groups and goals deemed desirable by nurses. Means for attaining those ends are available to man in varying degrees. They are identified as health-seeking and coping behaviors (mechanisms) actively employed by man in his efforts to attain or retain optimal health and function, to overcome threats to health, and to cope with crises encountered during his development and decline and at the time of death. Intervening variables (including diagnostic and therapeutic procedures) cause alteration in physiological, psychological, and social mechanisms typically available to individuals and to groups.

The nurses's responsibilities include *compensating* for man's health-seeking behaviors in some circumstances, and in others, altering, maintaining, or enhancing them through use of nursing strategies appropriate to each unique nursing situation. Those nursing strategies include use of a variety of means and modalities, including direct, personal interactions and transactions and a variety of nursing techniques, devices, and technological aids. They include

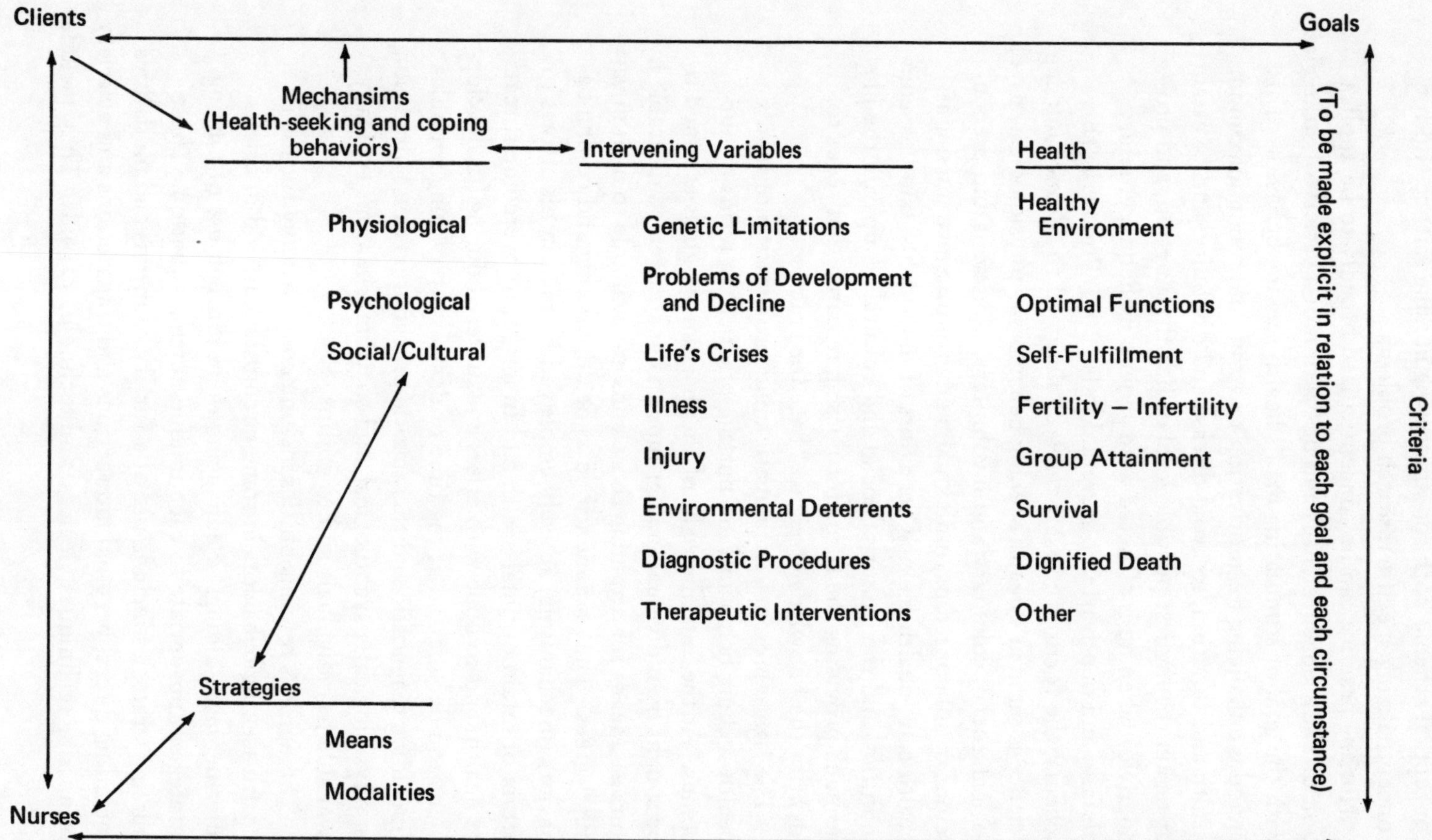

Figure. A paradigm for conceptualizing nursing research.

observing, evaluating, communicating, ministering, teaching, counseling, motivating, nurturing, and inspiring.

Within this conceptualization the nurse professional recognizes the characteristic independence and interdependence of man and his occasional dependence; the practitioner envisions nursing practice to be the use of strategies that maximize each person's unique potential for self-actualization as it relates to attaining health and function, as well as strategies that promote the public's health.

Nursing research cast in this conceptual scheme focuses on study of the behavior of individuals and groups to be served by professionals. It assumes inherent and innate capabilities in man, some of which may be latent; it also assumes that some capabilities must be actualized through guided learning and recognizes potentials and limitations in capacities that are genetically and environmentally determined. It assumes that self-actualization is possible and desirable through maximizing each individual's inherent capacities and his capacity to change goals and behavior through learning. It assumes that the goal of nurses is to utilize knowledge of man relevant to his health-seeking behaviors artfully and skillfully through use of nursing strategies that assist him in realizing his maximum potential as it relates to wellness and optimal function.

Much knowledge is needed about man's "typical" health-seeking behaviors and about coping behaviors as they are manifested during illness, injury, deprivations, change in life-style, life crises, and impending death. Knowledge is also needed about group behavior (and its motivation) as it relates to promotion of community health and dealing with environmental health hazards.

Much needs to be known also about the relative efficacy of nursing interventions and modalities and the timing and style of their implementation. It is appropriate to test through systematic inquiry the relative efficacy of these strategies that represent the gamut of nursing practices, just as it is appropriate to test the relative efficacy of extant dental, educational, engineering, or medical strategies, techniques, and devices at any point in time.

This approach for conceptualizing nursing (and research through which knowledge is generated) requires enunciation and consensual validation of specific, desired goals and explication of statements concerning relationships between means and ends. Knowledge unique to the profession of nursing is that which will emerge as nursing science when sufficient systematic inquiry is conducted to infirm or confirm explicitly stated relationships between identified means and desired ends.

Advancement of nursing knowledge can be approached inductively through empirical inquiry or deductively through tests of postulated theory, as can advancement of knowledge in any intellectual discipline. Some illustrations of nursing research utilizing both approaches to adding to the knowledge base for nursing practice demonstrate the practicality of approaches that conceptualize nursing research in terms of knowledge needed to attain explicit goals.

Empirical study of man's health-seeking behaviors can reveal how each individual's capacities are affected by genetic inadequacies, environmental and cultural factors, injury, pathology, maturation and decline, and life's crises; replicated studies focusing on the health-seeking behaviors of individuals and groups under varied circumstances will permit valid generalizations about the health-seeking behaviors of man in general. Hypothetical constructs about the health-seeking behaviors of individuals (and groups) can and should be explicated and tested repeatedly with a view toward inductively developing theories of use to nurses in practice [21]. After repeated test and verification, such theoretical constructs become verified objective knowledge (science) basic to the practice of nursing.

The classic study done by Tudor [22] provides one illustration of careful documentation of human behavior in a reasonably controlled natural setting. Her work involved repeated observations of patients manifesting behavioral aberrations in a nursing practice setting to obtain data for verification of the hypothesis that withdrawal behavior on the part of staff enhances the pathological withdrawal behavior of patients. Deliberately planned interventions directed toward reducing staff-patient reciprocal withdrawal were tested for their efficacy in promoting social behavior deemed desirable on the part of the patients. Theoretical notions concerning the social context within which care is given were advanced. Tudor's pioneer work also made a substantial methodological contribution to inquiry in nursing.

Beginning with interest in aberrant behavior ostensibly associated with the variable of reduction in sensory stimulation, called sensory deprivation, Jackson and his associates have been involved in several empirical investigations seeking to gain knowledge about the consequences of such deprivation. In a series of clinical studies of patients who experienced social isolation and visual and auditory impairment, evidence was obtained to document the fact that such patients report (and staff verify) that they have a wide variety of perceptual experiences [10]. Causal factors and the clinical significance of experiences purportedly associated with altered stimulation have, however, not yet been established [9]. This work has contributed to the generation of theoretical notions about the ranges of "normal" and the amounts and typical patterns of stimulation required by persons that may be found, with future research, to be optimal for their well-being.

A series of investigations undertaken by proponents of Rogers' [18] conceptual scheme have made significant contributions to the advancement of nursing knowledge. Two dealing with problems of human stimulation are briefly described here.

Rogers postulates a single conceptual model of man that provides a framework for nursing inquiry. According to her scheme, man is a unified system that cannot be understood except in his wholeness and in the complementarity of his relationship to his environment. Thus for Rogers [19], the notion of studying man's social behavior, his physiological behavior, or his psychological behavior would be inappropriate for the investigator who seeks to advance nursing science.

Utilizing the conceptual framework appropriate to the theoretical notion that the human organism represents an energy field in constant motion and interaction with his environment, Porter [17] tested the hypotheses that increases in the growth and development of infants (as evidenced by gains in weight and length, motor behavior, language behavior, adaptive behavior, and personal-social behavior) could be significantly enhanced by planned, passive exercises. It was predicted that the dynamic changes theoretically ongoing in the human energy field would be accelerated by periodic, passive kinesthetic stimulation. The experimental variable consisted of cycling exercises of the infants' upper and lower extremities, twice daily for two five-minute periods, alternating with two five-minute rest periods. The exercise regime was continuous over six days each week for a period of two months. The findings supported the hypothesis and consequently added credence to the theoretical formulation that provided the conceptual framework for Porter's study.

Using a conceptual model that postulates the value of imprinting and patterned sensory stimulation (in contrast to sensory deprivation) for the growth and development of premature infants, Katz [12] designed research to determine the effect of patterned stimulation on behavior development in incubated infants. The patterned stimulation provided for each infant was a recording of the mother's voice played periodically each day for infants from their fifth day of life until each infant reached a gestational age of 252 days. A control group of infants did not receive this stimulation. The findings supported the hypothesis that infants who had had the auditory stimulation demonstrated significantly greater maturational development and auditory and visual response and were less irritable than those who served as controls. Knowledge about the environmental circumstances that enhance the health status of premature infants was advanced by Katz's research, research that was guided by a conceptual framework derived from an explicated theory of man.

SUMMARY

It is the thesis of this chapter that all systematic inquiry requires a conceptual framework that serves as a guide to observations and as a scheme for interpreting and organizing knowledge that derives therefrom. The assumption was made that nursing as a learned practice profession has a unique body of knowledge that must be continuously advanced and restructured. Several conceptual models for guiding systematic inquiry (and for organizing knowledge of the field) were discussed.

No one conceptual model is appropriate for all research, inasmuch as knowledge derived from research serves several purposes. The conceptual model selected should be commensurate with the intent of the investigator.

REFERENCES

1. Barker, K. N., Kimbrough, W. W., and Heller, W. M. *A Study of Medication Errors in a Hospital.* Fayetteville: University of Arkansas, 1966.
2. Boskoff, A. Process-orientation in sociological theory and research: Untasted old wine in slightly used bottles. *Social Forces* 50:1–12, 1971.
3. Committee for the Study of Nursing Education. *Nursing and Nursing Education in the United States.* Report of the Committee for the Study of Nursing Education and Report of a Survey by Josephine Goldmark. New York: Macmillan, 1923, pp. 56–96.
4. Churchman, C. W. *The Systems Approach.* New York: Delacorte, 1968.
5. Glaser, B., and Strauss, A. *Awareness of Dying.* Chicago: Aldine, 1965.
6. Hallstrom, B. J. Utilization of nursing personnel: A task-specific approach. *Nursing Outlook* 19:664–667, 1971.
7. Hardy, J. D., Wolff, H. G., and Goodell, H. *Pain Sensations and Reactions.* New York: Hafner, 1967.
8. Ibid., pp. 261–306, 379–392.
9. Jackson, C. W., Jr., and Ellis, R. Sensory deprivation as a field of study. *Nursing Research,* 20:46–54, 1971.
10. Jackson, C. W., Jr., and O'Neil, M. Experiences Associated with Sensory Deprivation for Patients Having Eye Surgery. In J. E. Jeffries (Ed.), *Patients with Sensory Disturbances – Implications for Nursing Practice and Research.* Columbus, Ohio: Ross Laboratories, 1966.
11. Johns, E., and Pfefferkorn, B. *An Activity Analysis of Nursing.* New York: Committee on the Grading of Nursing Schools, 1934.
12. Katz, V. Auditory stimulation and developmental behavior of the premature infant. *Nursing Research* 20:196–201, 1971.
13. Lewis, C. E., and Resnik, B. A. Nurse clinics and progressive ambulatory care. *New England Journal of Medicine* 277:1236–1241, 1967.
14. Nadler, G. *Work Systems Design: The IDEALS Concept.* Homewood, Ill.: Richard D. Irwin, Inc., 1967.
15. Newton, M. E., Hunt, W. E., McDowell, W. E., and Hanken, A. F. *A Study of Nurse Action in Relief of Pain.* Columbus, Ohio: The Ohio State University Research Foundation, 1964.
16. *Nurse Utilization: A Patient Care Systems Project.* A Report of the Wisconsin Regional Medical Program, Inc., under the auspices of the University of Wisconsin–Milwaukee School of Nursing, 1972.
17. Porter, L. S. The impact of physical-physiological activity on infants' growth and development. *Nursing Research* 21:210–219, 1972.
18. Rogers, M. E. *An Introduction to the Theoretical Basis of Nursing.* Philadelphia: Davis, 1970.
19. Rogers, M. E. The Ph.D. in Nursing. In *Future Directions of Doctoral Education for Nurses.* Washington, D.C.: United States Government Printing Office, 1971. Department of Health, Education, and Welfare, Publication Number (NIH) 72–82.
20. Schlotfeldt, R. M. Nursing in health care. *Nursing Outlook* 20:245–246, 1972.

21. Schlotfeldt, R. M. The significance of empirical research for nursing. *Nursing Research* 20:140–142, 1971.
22. Tudor, G. E. A sociopsychiatric nursing approach to intervention in a problem of mutual withdrawal on a mental hospital ward. *Perspectives in Psychiatric Care* 8:11–35, 1970. (Reprinted from *Psychiatry* 15:193–217, 1952.)
23. Yankauer, A., Connelly, J. P., and Feldman, J. J. Pediatric practice in the United States – with special attention to utilization of allied health worker services. *Pediatrics* 45:521–550, 1970.
24. Zborowski, M. Cultural components in responses to pain. *Journal of Social Issues* 8(4):16–30, 1952.

A Process for Developing Concepts for Nursing through Research

Imogene M. King

2

HUMAN beings are bombarded with a multitude of facts in their daily lives through concrete sensory experiences. From these concrete experiences, man has an ability to form concepts, which are abstractions that give meaning to his world of reality. The knowledge explosion in the real world is a major problem confronting many professions and occupations in the 1970s. Increased knowledge from research in various fields of inquiry continues to be disseminated in large quantities and sometimes in fragmented bits and pieces of information. One approach to coping with these problems in a field such as nursing is the development of concepts and theories. Understanding theoretical concepts that form the foundations of nursing will help nurses use scientific knowledge in the performance of their functions.

Theory represents reality. Sets of concepts found in theories are abstractions that explain real-world phenomena. Some understanding of the human process of knowing, of the process of concept development generally and concept development for nursing specifically, is an essential part of the scientific study of nursing practice. The mutual interdependence of observation (empirical facts) and theory (concepts) is demonstrated in research. One approach to concept development and theory construction through research is presented in this chapter. On the basis of the guidelines used here, you may become aware of the process you use for developing concepts relevant for nursing.

This chapter will attempt to explain a deductive-inductive process of thinking about nursing and will begin with some notions of the relevance to nursing of concept development through research.

RELEVANCE OF CONCEPT DEVELOPMENT FOR NURSING

The beginning of scientific activity consists in describing, classifying, and correlating phenomena. Nurses have engaged in these activities for many years and have collected masses of data in the process of giving nursing care. The problem has been that once specific concrete data are collected and used by nurses, they are lost for future analysis. In other words, the concepts used by individuals have not always been made explicit so that they may be tested and verified in the empirical world of nursing.

Direct observation has been a primary function of nurses for centuries. Nurses collect voluminous data in their daily activities to gain immediate factual information to plan and give nursing care. They have been trained to make observations and to measure selected physiological and behavioral parameters of human beings to answer immediate questions. Research training in nonparticipant and participant observations, however, has been limited in initial programs that prepare practitioners. Some recent changes in undergraduate programs have included these skills. Ways must be discovered to marshal the observations and measurements made by nurses to answer scientific questions through systematic investigation of empirical problems. In this way, then, concepts and theories can be tested empirically by use of appropriate scientific procedures and thus give meaning to one's picture of reality in nursing situations.

Some of the more recent publications by nurses [5, 15] in the 1970s advocated the use of a conceptual framework to guide empirical observations, both in conducting research in nursing and in developing curriculums for teaching professional practice to students in higher education. In 1952, Peplau [14] presented interpersonal relations as a theoretical position in nursing. This was one of the first conceptual frameworks in modern nursing, although Nightingale [12] had implied one by choosing to write about concepts such as health, illness, environment, and nutrition.

A generic orientation as to what nursing is; what decisions nurses are required to make; what reactions, interactions, and transactions are occurring in nursing situations that improve health states or health outcomes – all are essential factors to be considered in scientific investigations in nursing. Theoretical formulations facilitate the process for deriving specific hypotheses to test through research.

In addition, theoretical positions identify some fundamental concepts relevant for nursing practice. As theories for nursing continue to be formulated and tested, relationships from a multitude of fragmented bits of information will be identified and will give the profession a common language of concepts. Nurses must exploit theoretical ideas by empirical observations to clarify the designs of inquiry into the nature of practice.

As in any other field of study, inquiry into nursing requires a cadre of interested and qualified nurses to search for knowledge through descriptions, classifications, and explanations of events, persons, and situations. The real-life situations in nursing provide a major source of ideas for formulating concepts that, when defined, can be verified. Descriptive data collected systematically are a source of concepts. In contrast, one may identify and develop concepts and then verify them empirically. Descriptions of patterns of behavior provide a wealth of information from which nurses conducting research can continue to formulate and test hypotheses.

It must be emphasized that no matter how refined the methodology and data collection instruments, the research will have little meaning for building knowledge for use by nurses unless the concepts selected have some relationship to nursing practice. Communicating findings in writing to other nurses helps one continue to gain in exactness and clarity. In Bacon's essay "Of Studies" he stated: "Reading maketh a full man; conference a ready man; and writing an exact man" [1]. As scientific knowledge in a subject such as nursing is increased through research and the findings are communicated and utilized, concepts in nursing will be modified.

The nature of the human process for knowing one's external environment is more than an intellectual exercise; it is an integral part of every human being. The process of acquiring knowledge is a common characteristic of man. Thus a conscious awareness of the way we develop concepts that give us knowledge about our environment lays the groundwork for understanding how scientific concepts are developed and verified in nursing through research. The major difference between the acquisition of everyday knowledge and of scientific knowledge is that the latter is acquired through a systematically controlled research process. However, understanding concept development generally is essential for identifying ideas specifically for nursing and for testing them through research.

The Nature of Concepts

Scientists have made many investigations of processes through which individuals categorize sense data. Their findings have indicated that the nervous system is a human data processing system. Through perception, a mental faculty, information is processed and ideas are abstracted from the real world. Perception is referred to as a data reduction system.

We frequently talk about objects and events in terms of the wholes and the parts, the global and the specific, and the universal and the particular. In so doing we are looking for some kind of order in the information we receive about our world through our sensory experiences. Concepts are abstract ideas that give meaning to concrete sensory experiences.

Concepts As a Way of Knowing

Man functions in an external environment that continually bombards him with multiple stimuli. These stimuli activate nerve impulses in the sense organs that are sent to the brain via the neural network of the nervous system. Association pathways in the brain and memory (stored data) contribute to the process of gaining knowledge. According to Konorski [11], the cognitive or gnostic system is concerned with perceptions and behavior. Through the process of perception, the external world is analyzed. Information is processed by selecting certain stimuli from all the stimuli presented, by categorizing, or classifying, the data received, and by organizing them within a relevant framework of past experience and past and present knowledge.

In the process of growth and development through the life cycle, human beings are provided a wide range of sensory experiences. These experiences offer the raw materials whereby human beings perceive objects, persons, and events in the external environment. These experiences put individuals in direct contact with the outside world through taste, touch, smell, sound, and sight. Thus, *one element in the process of developing concepts is sensory perception.*

From perceptions, individuals form *concepts* that give meaning to a wide variety of concrete sense data by naming things. A *concept* is defined here as an abstract idea or a mental image formed by generalizations from specific sensory experiences. Figure 2-1 is a representation of the accumulation of sensory experiences into a concept. *Naming* is a second element in the process of forming concepts. In naming, we use verbal symbols that signify objects or persons. Naming things provides a way of discovering that there are similarities and differences in our sensory perceptions.

When a new object is perceived as different from all other objects, or as similar to some other objects, a process of discrimination or differentiation occurs. In this *process of differentiation,* individuals seek common attributes in their experiences. This results in the organization of sensory data into categories or groupings of experiences.

An example of this process can be seen when one observes a child exploring the chairs in his home. He touches some; he sits on others. He discovers the specific attributes of chairs – they have legs, seats, are soft or hard, straight, rocking, or swivel type, and so on. He is perceiving many chairs from concrete experiences with a variety of sizes, shapes, and colors. He begins to differentiate between types of chairs in the living room and those in the dining room. When he says "This is a lawn chair for the patio," he has begun to label or name the chairs and differentiate their use. Any object he observes or uses in the future that resembles those he has experienced will be tested against his idea of chair and the common attributes he categorizes as *chair.* He has formed a concept of chair.

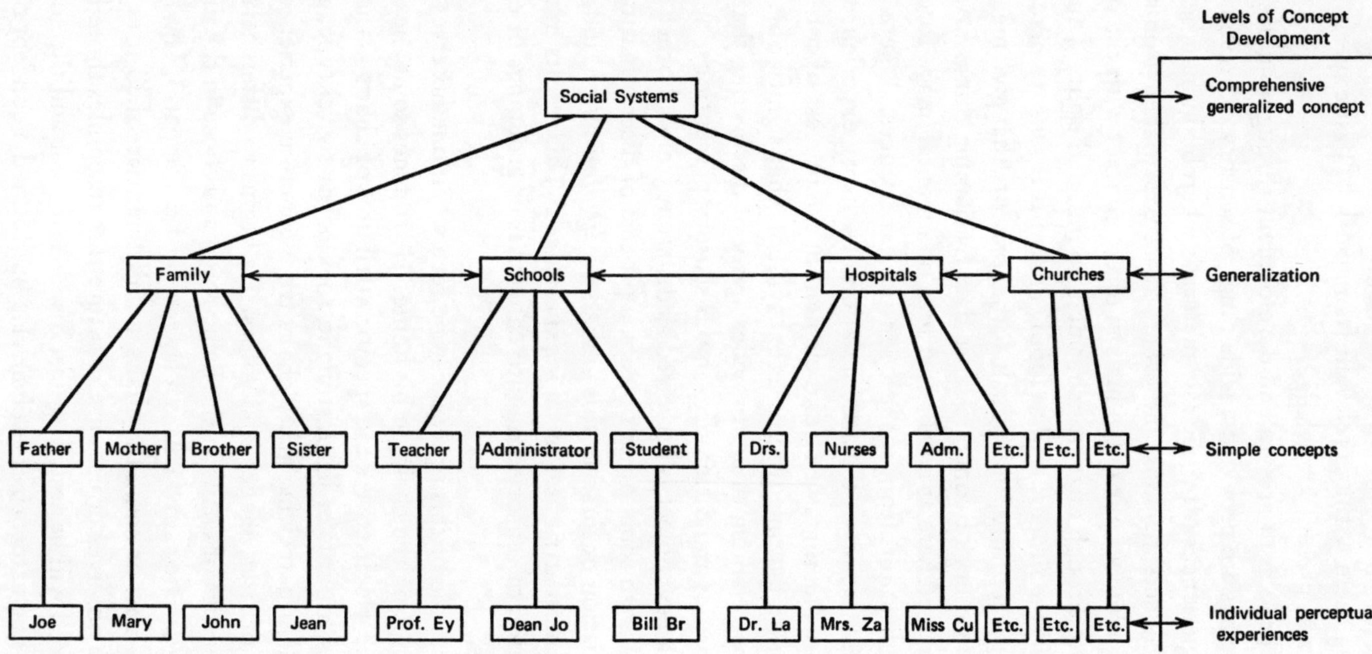

Fig. 2-1. A way of describing levels of conceptualization from concrete experiences to abstract generalizations. (From King [6].)

This process, which begins with sensory perceptions and moves to naming things, to differentiation and categorization of sensory experiences, and forming generalizations about one's environment, is the way human beings develop concepts.

A concept represents essential elements that an object has in common with others of the same class. A concept *dog,* for example, is not like an image of an individual dog, limited to the white poodle lying at your feet. On the contrary, it represents what is common to all dogs and may be applied to each and every dog. Any concept, then, is universal in that it represents certain common elements that can be applied to all in a class. A concept is an intellectual means of representing multiple concrete objects and things. If you and I express verbally to each other our individual concepts of weather, some common elements such as rain, snow, and sleet would be terms we would use to describe our concept. If you said "Sunshine in too great amounts may cause skin blemishes," and I said "I like cold weather because it is invigorating," these statements indicate some differences in our concepts of weather.

In the act of knowing about one's environment, perception helps us gain an awareness of persons, objects, and events in our world. Each individual knows his environment on the basis of his perceptions of reality. Concepts, however, are the generalized abstractions that give meaning to concrete experiences. Thus your concept of weather and mine are similar in common attributes but different because of our individual perceptual experiences. My conception of the moon and the astronauts' conception are different largely because of my lack of scientific knowledge and experience. My conception of the moon is different from what it was in 1960 because the explorations of the moon since then have given me new information about it. As one gains information and new facts, one's concepts are modified or become more comprehensive.

A prelude to the use of a scientific process has been presented here. A conscious awareness of a human process of knowing, a way of thinking, is essential for identifying concepts relevant for nursing. When one understands how man acquires information about the world and utilizes categories to conceptualize it, the identification and development of concepts for nursing are facilitated. Through research into the nature of nursing practice, new knowledge or new relationships among concepts will be discovered. These scientific concepts developed through research in nursing are defined as generalizations formulated from scientific inquiry.

Why this emphasis on concepts in nursing in the 1970s? Concepts serve several functions in nursing. One is to help us cope with the information explosion in a technological society, and another is to guide nurses in their research efforts to develop theories for nursing. Concepts help nurses retain knowledge for use in nursing practice.

FUNCTIONS OF CONCEPTS

Language is an instrument through which people communicate with one another. One of the functions of language is to maintain a correspondence with one's experience. It follows that words and their meaning influence the identification and development of concepts relevant for nursing. Analysis of the meaning of terms must therefore focus on the particular contexts in which they are used. Many concepts of a theoretical nature relate only indirectly to experiences. Their meaning in experience depends on the context of the immediate situation. So to find what concepts mean, we have to examine how to apply them. One analyzes a concept by attempting to get at its use. One analyzes the structure in terms of functions.

Empirical inquiry into the nature of nursing necessitates a selection of concepts to guide the collection and analysis of data. Concepts serve as building blocks in theory development. Kaplan [3] explained that "to find what a scientific concept means, examine how you apply it, or how you apply other concepts related to it. But what else has anyone ever done? Indeed, what else is there to do?" He noted, too, that "the function of scientific concepts is to mark the categories which will tell us more about our subject matter than any other categorial sets" [4]. The concept of system, for example, marks off categories such as structure, function, roles, and processes that guide the researcher in delineating the problem he wishes to study. The concepts in a theory are the categories. A concept is an organization of reference points. As *cells are units of the body, concepts are units of the mind* by which individuals store past experiences in the memory. Words are the verbal symbols used to explain events and things in our environment and relationships to past experiences. As Northrop stated:

A theory of any kind, whether scientific or philosophic, is a body of propositions, and a body of propositions is a set of concepts. Concepts fall into different types according to the different sources of their meaning. . . . A concept is a term to which a meaning has been assigned [13].

The road to scientific inquiry is paved with concepts. Sets of concepts formally stated in a body of propositions that are interrelated provide theoretical frameworks in any empirical science. These frameworks give us pathways to explore; they tell us what to observe.

Concepts give us the starting point in the journey to search for knowledge. Concepts give us the means of travel by *specifying operations* essential *for observing variables* along the roads. Concepts help us to arrive deductively at new roads or to resurface or renovate old roads. Thus the research process to test a concept may be initiated when there is a question to be answered, a principle to be demonstrated, or a problem to be solved.

DEVELOPING CONCEPTS FOR NURSING – A PROCESS

Where do we find concepts for nursing? Ideas come from a variety of sources, such as inferences from one's observations, discussions with colleagues, the literature in nursing and related fields of study, and deductions from theories. Ideas do not come in a vacuum-packed container but are creations of each human being as he explains his world. Ideas are the product of our language and culture and of our being nurses and thus immersed in a particular field with its values, concepts, and skills applied in real-world situations.

Developing concepts for nursing through research is an ongoing dynamic process. Among other things it involves scientific investigation into the nature of nursing. Moreover, it is a scientific process through which nurses discover new insights to expand knowledge and also is a way of thinking about and studying nursing in a conscious, deliberative, and systematic way. The essence of this process involves a series of inductions and deductions about specific ideas relevant for nursing practice.

The *inductive process* is a mental act of arriving at some generalizations from organized masses of data. For example, you have been systematically collecting and recording the data of direct observations of nurse-patient interactions over a specified period of time. In your analysis of these data you discover patterns of behavior that indicate when transactions have occurred between the nurse and each patient. This is induction, which is proceeding from specific observed data to formulating a general concept about what the nursing process is, such as, "The nursing process is a series of interactions that may or may not result in transactions." The inductive process begins with an operational definition of the concept. This is followed by observations, descriptions, and classification of facts relevant to the concept. From these concrete data, concepts are verified in the real world.

The *deductive process* is a mental act of proposing hypothetico-deductive propositions with minimal empirical evidence. The investigator speculates as to the logical relationships among the propositions. Deductive formulations guide empirical investigations. For example, my general proposition is that nursing is a process of action, reaction, and interaction, and that at some point in the future (minutes, days, weeks) the nurse and patient reach a transaction about the goal to be achieved in the situation. When the transactions occur, there will be perceptual accuracy by nurse and patient. When transactions do not occur, incongruence in nurse-patient perceptions will be observable in their presenting behaviors. In order to verify these propositions, direct observations of nurse-patient interactions are made in a systematic way over time to gather descriptive data from which specific hypotheses may be formulated to test in the real world. The deductive process, in which concepts in the problem are explained or verified in data collected, uses formal logic and mathematics in its analysis. Data produced by deductive theory are used to refine or modify it.

The research process, a combination of deduction and induction, is used in any scientific inquiry into the nature of things. Developing concepts for nursing gives one a purpose or objective to be achieved through research. The first element in the research process is the statement, limitation, and analysis of the problem, or formulation of the question(s). A second element in the process is to determine the ways in which empirical data can be objectively and systematically gathered. Attention is given to data collection and to tools and techniques that will in fact help gather data. A third element is to determine the ways to analyze the data collected and statistics give us this assistance. A fourth element is the interpretation of the facts gathered. This process is apparent as one reads published research.

The use of theory, concepts, deductive logic, and inductive observations and experimentations cannot be overemphasized in a discussion of a process of inquiry into the nature of nursing. This is a process whereby concepts are identified, developed, tested, and verified in an empirical science such as nursing.

The process of developing concepts for nursing through research is a continuous activity of inquiry whereby nurses continue to build a body of knowledge for use by practitioners. In the process of categorizing bits and pieces of information from many specific experiences, the researcher is engaging in other processes or cognitive operations, namely, thinking, judging, reasoning, and making inferences.

Studies of real nursing situations that describe patterns of behaviors of organisms in their natural states are essential for developing concepts and theories. The interpersonal laboratory in which nurses function daily provides a setting for naturalistic descriptive studies. Collection of data through direct observations of behaviors that naturally occur over time is not without problems. If the process of observation is to produce data that can be handled in a scientific manner, the observations must be made for a specific purpose, be done systematically, and be controlled by the observer. It is purposiveness and control that differentiates scientific observations from everyday perceptual experiences. Systematic observations are preceded by a clear statement of a problem to be studied and the purpose of the study.

It must be emphasized that any scientific inquiry into nursing should indicate its conceptual system, because the system not only serves as a guide to research but also provides a framework for building a body of knowledge. Scientific concepts provide categories in the subject to be studied. Verification is made possible when definitions of the concepts are derived from systematic investigations.

VERIFICATION OF CONCEPTS IN NURSING THROUGH RESEARCH

Individuals make inferences and verify their ideas continuously. A simple example is a person observing that a coin is silver and about ½ inch in diameter and putting these two perceptions together and naming it a dime. The category is money. By the process of deduction, one identifies the purpose for a dime and tests this in reality by purchasing something with the money.

Verification of scientific concepts through research is not so simple. Theorists have implied that a process of verification of concepts indicates gradations, such as high, average, low degree of confirmation of concept in empirical evidence. Concepts are derived by each person from his own experiences and are constantly tested and changed from experiences. Bronowski had this to say:

> . . . the place of experience is to test and correct the concept. The test is, Will the concept work? Does it give an unforced unity to the experience of men? Does the concept make life orderly, not by edict but in fact? [2]

Demonstration of Use of a Process

My personal approach to synthesizing knowledge for nursing was to use data and information available from research in nursing and related fields and from my 25 years in active practice, teaching, and research. From all the knowledge available, a theoretical framework relevant for nursing was formulated. The first step in the process was the completion of an extensive review of published research in nursing and related behavioral sciences, looking for recurring ideas or for concepts that were undergoing verification through systematic investigation. A series of questions guided this review of literature. These questions were formulated specifically to identify the nature of nursing. They were:

1. What is the nursing act?
2. What is the nursing process?
3. What is the goal of nursing?
4. Who are nurses, and how are they educated for practice?
5. How and where is nursing practiced?
6. Who needs nursing in this society?

A search of the literature in nursing and other behavioral science fields, discussion with colleagues, attendance at numerous conferences, inductive and deductive reasoning, and some critical thinking about the information gathered, led me to formulate my own theoretical framework [7].

My general systems theory consists of four major concepts that are interrelated and can be found in any human situation and therefore in any nursing situation. These major concepts cut across disciplinary lines and are applicable in any field of inquiry that involves interaction of human beings to achieve purposes and goals. Figure 2-2 is a diagram of my systems framework.

Any phenomenon called systems has a goal. *Health*, one of the major concepts in my theoretical framework, is the goal for nursing. Two of the four concepts that focus on the dynamics of nursing, *perception* and *interpersonal relations*, guided me to relate research findings about these two ideas to the *nursing process*. The nursing process is defined as a series of acts that connote action, reaction, interaction, and transaction between nurse and health client [8]. The fourth concept in the framework is *social systems*, since nurses, doctors, patients, health clients, and families grow and develop within social organizations that involve roles, position, and status. Health is the goal of the system; perception is a basic concept in the *personal or self system;* interpersonal relations is a basic concept in the *interpersonal system;* and social organization is a basic concept in *social systems.*

These four comprehensive generalized concepts guided me to

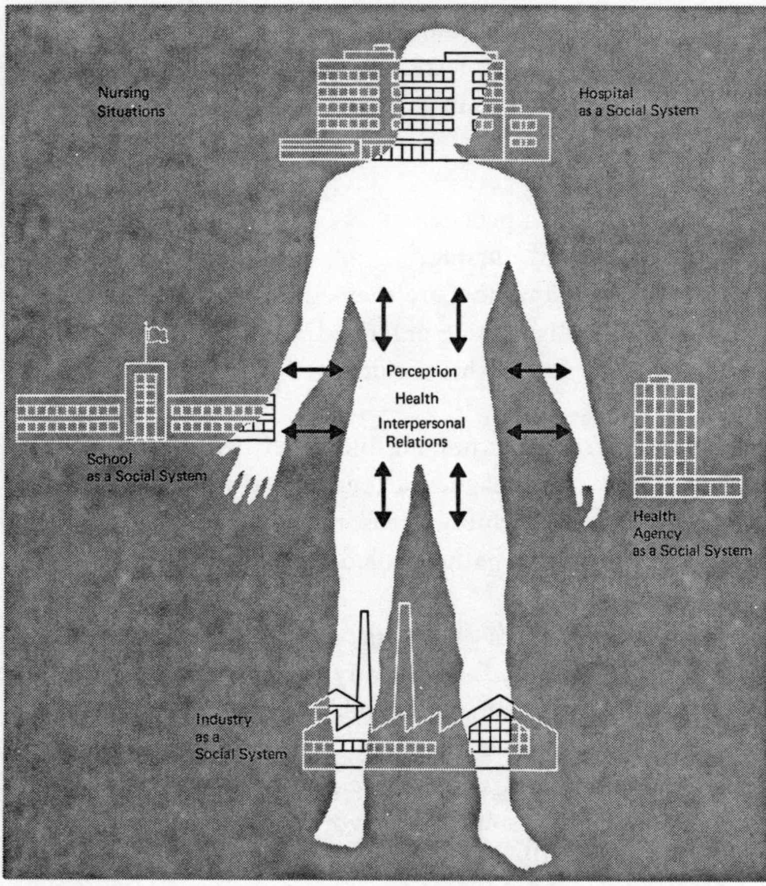

Fig. 2-2. Theoretical framework with the four major concepts. Theoretical framework: personal systems, interpersonal systems, social systems. Four major concepts: health as the goal of the systems; perception – personal systems; interpersonal relations – interpersonal systems; social organization – social systems. (Adapted from King [9].)

formulate a working definition for nursing process. My purpose for conducting research is to attempt to verify my concept of nursing process, which is the core of nursing.

The first step in the process of formulating a program of research to verify concepts in my theoretical framework in natural nursing situations was to ask some questions about nursing for which I had no answers. These questions guided me to specific studies in nursing to determine if any common ideas had been developed. Some of the concepts have been sparsely tested, and there was no evidence of verification through similar research methodology and techniques.

The next step in the process leading to design of a systematic study of the nursing process to verify the concept as I have defined it is to formulate some hypotheses. My hunch is that in many nursing situations, the perceptions of the nurse and the perceptions of the health client are incongruent; there is disagreement as to goals to be achieved in specific nursing situations; there is disagreement as to the means to be used to achieve goals. Within the nurse-client interaction process, it is further hypothesized that when nurse and client through one or more interactions arrive at a transaction (mutually agreed-upon goals), health outcomes for the client will be improved. What is the next step in the process?

A model [10] for studying the human process of establishing interpersonal relationships serves as the structure to conceptualize a way to study the nursing process. Figure 2-3 presents such a model. This model indicates that the vehicle for collecting data

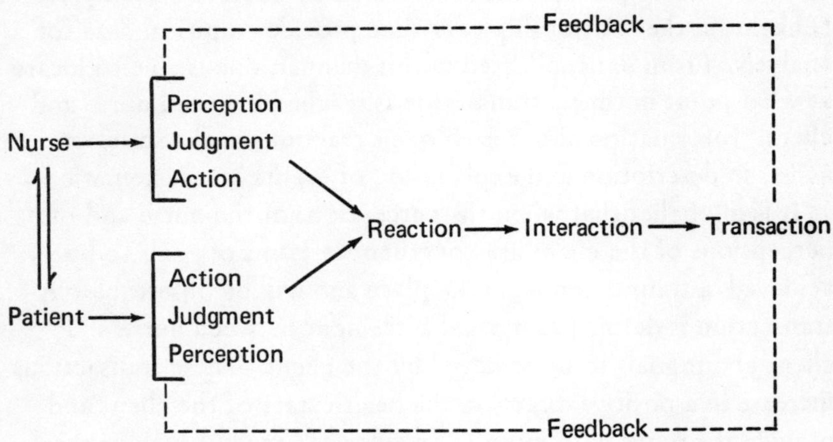

Fig. 2-3. A model for studying the nursing process (From King [10].)

about nursing process is through direct observations of nurse-client interactions. Collecting information about nurse and health client in a specific situation over time through direct observations of verbal and nonverbal behavior will provide data that describe and classify phenomena in the interactions. An assumption is made that inferences can be drawn about the client's reactions to the situation and events and persons in it, as well as transactions that may come about through the interactions. These interactions over time are shown in Figure 2-4. Time 1, 2, 3, . . . n may be seconds, minutes, hours, and days, depending on the length of the interaction and the intervals as defined in the research design.

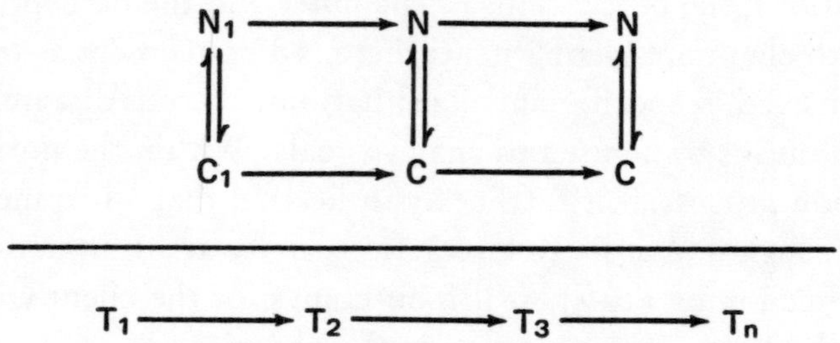

Fig. 2-4. **Nurse (*N*) and Client (*C*) interactions over time.**

Figure 2-4 shows, too, how a series of acts of two interacting individuals whose perceptions are inferred by observing each person's behavior in the relationship over time provide empirical data for analysis. From data collected in this manner, one is able to locate at what point in time a transaction is reached between nurse and client. Information about each one's reactions in the situation assists in description and explanation of events in a systematic way.

It is my belief that when the perceptions of the nurse and the perceptions of the client are congruent in terms of goals to be achieved, a transaction will take place and will be observable. A transaction is defined as mutual agreement between nurse and client about goals to be achieved by the client. These transactions increase in a positive direction the health state of the client and provide the nurse with more knowledge of human behavior that may be useful at some future time. In other words, there is growth in a positive direction for both nurse and client. Peplau [14] discussed the idea of positive growth in nurse-client relationships in the 1950s in her interpersonal relations theory for nursing. If nurses continue to verify this concept through further research, some generalizations may be made about the nursing process.

A third element in the process of verifying concepts through research is the selection of a sample or of situations in which the data will be collected. As previously mentioned, the process of inquiry for developing concepts requires data collection techniques, procedures, and statistics that are appropriate for the problem. My research program has been planned to gather descriptive data about my theoretical concept of nursing. Those descriptive data will generate hypotheses to test my theoretical concept. Tentatively, my plan is to select one sample of adult individuals hospitalized for surgical intervention and a second sample of adults hospitalized for therapy in an acute crisis, such as a sudden heart attack. Variables such as age, sex, and surgical procedure will be controlled in the first sample. Variables such as age, sex, and medical regimen for acute crises therapy will be controlled in the second sample. The nonparticipant direct observation technique will be utilized to collect all information. These will be continuous observations of all interactions between nurse and patient from admission through discharge from the hospital. The focus of data collection is to describe interactions between $N_{1 \ldots n}$ (nurse) and $P_{1 \ldots p}$ (patient) over the time period of the hospitalization event, rather than on securing large samples of patients, and to analyze interactions to determine the transactions or goals in the situation. At this point in the process, I would seek out a statistician for assistance in the kind of statistical measures that would be appropriate for use with the kind of data being collected and the hypotheses to be tested.

The next step in the process is to collect data and use the statistical procedures agreed on with the statistician for analysis. Interpretations are made from the data that indicate either (1) confirmation or rejection of the hypotheses, or (2) verification of the concept that nursing is a process of action, reaction, interaction, and transaction that leads to positive health outcomes, or (3) both. The process of deduction and induction continues because it is an ongoing dynamic process, since the findings of one study raise more questions to be researched.

This is a brief overview of how one nurse identified and developed basic concepts she perceived as relevant for nursing. Currently, a research program is being formulated to describe transactions in natural nursing situations from which hypotheses can be generated to test one theoretical concept in nursing. The concepts of a theory that have not been verified in research become useless, and research that is not grounded in theory is sterile. The process described in this chapter is one way of thinking about and studying nursing practice.

Investigators now have available new techniques that are helpful in collecting and analyzing data. The computer, which can handle masses of data and analyze many variables in complex systems, has greatly lessened the task of data analysis. The videotape can record such events as nurse-patient-physician-family interactions in nursing situations. This technique preserves real-world data for analysis by one or more investigators for validity and reliability of observations. Simulations of events in natural situations is another approach being used to study health care systems and nursing. One example is the use of models (life sized) to test for cardiopulmonary resuscitation.

These new approaches to observation have enabled reproducibility of situations, as well as specificity and standardization of observation procedures, alleviating the difficulties of investigators who are attempting to verify the findings of others.

One of the goals of research in nursing is to explain natural phenomena and to use the knowledge from research to improve the health care of people. The processes of perception, conception, inductive and deductive reasoning, and critical thinking in designing research to test hypotheses and verify relevant concepts will help nurses achieve this end. The end of theoretical knowledge is its usefulness in the practical realm of action – the real world of nursing practice.

In conclusion, searching for scientific knowledge in the field of nursing is an ongoing dynamic process of continuous identification, development, and verification of relevant concepts.

REFERENCES

1. Bacon, F. Of Studies. In *Complete Essays of Francis Bacon* (introduction by P. H. Bailey). New York: Belmont, 1962, p. 151.
2. Bronowski, J. *Science and Human Values.* New York: Harper & Row, 1965, p. 41.
3. Kaplan, A. *A Conduct of Inquiry.* San Francisco: Chandler, 1964, p. 42.
4. Ibd., p. 52.
5. King, I. M. *Toward a Theory for Nursing.* New York: Wiley, 1971.
6. Ibid., p. 52.
7. Ibid., pp. 19–27.

8. Ibid., p. 25.
9. Ibid., p. 23.
10. Ibid., p. 92.
11. Konorski, J. *Integrative Activity of the Brain: An Interdisciplinary Approach.* Chicago: University of Chicago Press, 1967.
12. Nightingale, F. *Notes on Nursing: What It Is, and What It Is Not* (facsimile of 1st ed., London, 1859). Philadelphia: Lippincott, 1946.
13. Northrup, F. S. C. *The Logic of the Sciences and the Humanities.* Cleveland: Meridian, 1969, p. 82.
14. Peplau, H. E. *Interpersonal Relations in Nursing.* New York: G. P. Putnam's, 1952.
15. Rogers, M. E. *Introduction to the Theoretical Basis of Nursing.* Philadelphia: Davis, 1970.

Theory Development in Nursing

James Dickoff
Patricia James

3

PRELUDE

Ou sont les enfants?
Ils sont à l'église, mon père.
Pourquoi ne jouent pas les enfants?
Mais, mon père, ils jouent très bien à l'église. . . .

SOME REMINDERS TO A PURPOSE

This chapter makes no pretense of being a complete and systematic exposition. Such expositions, we have discovered, overwhelm readers. They become confused and contentious, and the aim of the communication – to make others able to go on with fruitful theory development – is unrealized. And so we confine ourselves here simply to assembling a few reminders to a purpose.

What prompts this approach? Experience with the unfruitfulness of other modes is surely a factor. Influential also in determining our tack is Ludwig Wittgenstein, a philosopher for the twentieth century. In his *Philosophical Investigations,* Wittgenstein [1] proposes that "The work of the philosopher consists in assembling reminders for a particular purpose." But why only reminders? Why not? A style that is obviously unelaborate, relatively unstructured, and suitably selective might be immediately more taking.

And so it may take up the reader. We would then achieve our aim as practical professionals. For philosophy, our profession, has as its unique task, to alter another's awareness.

But why bother to change a reader's outlook? To enable him to understand, that is, to enable him to go on. With what? With head and heart, so that he can *act* in producing what we as professionals see as a suitable good for the reader.

But reminders to what purpose? A dual one, at least. Again taking a cue from Wittgenstein, our purpose is in part a therapeutic one and so presupposes a diagnosis. Nursing, like certain tribes of philosophers, suffers from having put itself into foolishly unproductive postures. But does anyone knowingly adopt such a stance? This much seems clear: the force of old modes of thought – some of them indigenous to nursing, some inherited from without – overpowers the imagination. Things *must* be this way: there *cannot* be a new perspective. Said the four spinster daughters: "The Haydn quartet will be played this way because . . . because Papa did it this way." And does thinking escape such fetters? Wittgenstein speaks of thinking that is cramped and confined by "picture domination," of an imagination caught by the "trap of language," and of the need to let the fly out of the fly bottle. Do nurses think and talk about theory in such a way that theory becomes their fly bottle, their trap, their sanctuary?

Our purpose is more than therapeutic. Our reminders are to function as enablers for nurses. To be theoretical is, in our view, to be conceptual. More bluntly to theorize is to use language. Our aim is to enable nurses to use theory – and hence language – as a tool, not as a status badge or inhibitor.

To use language, however, is not merely to utter sounds, as in prayer, incantation, or recitation. Using language presupposes understanding of sounds. But what constitutes understanding? Again, following Wittgenstein, we suggest that understanding is perhaps best viewed as a capacity to go on. Understanding is not just seeing how things stand. Nor is understanding just contemplating the real, the true, the empirical, the clinical, or the linguistic. One understands when he has the capacity to be guided in activity by the articulated position, while yet in activity going beyond that position.

Taking understanding in this light liberates us from the inhibiting myths of complete explicitness, of an absolute order of things, or of given absolute simples. Nursing theorists are held captive by such myths. Consider Peplau [2], who seems to suggest that naming is a simple activity presupposed by other more complicated activities used in nursing conceptualization. But what makes an activity simple? Or, more basically, what is a "simple"? From one point of view, the more global activity may be "the simple": to do, to see, to grasp. To move to finer parts or atoms, to fracture the continuity into constitutive elements – *that* may be the more difficult. Pope, after all, said, "I lisp'd in numbers, for the numbers came." We purposely stress the ambiguity surrounding the word 'simple'. Simpleness is a relative notion, relative to purpose or else to an *already set pattern* of analysis.

Our usage throughout will be intentionally in contrast with a more pious use of language. The idols, though they are everywhere, are seen as deadweight only by those who dare a posture different from prayerful adoration. To break a fixation is our aim; to destroy a stance. Which one? The fixation that deifies the scientific while seeing the scientific as strongly opposed to the practical, the philosophical, and the "theoretical" – in the inventive sense of that word. The obsession that opposes the scientific to the value realm and to the realm of even professionally intersubjective preferences. Our reminders are aimed at creating a new posture, one that preserves for theoreticians the natural grace of common sense and professional practical sense. A stance that takes theory and research as an additive to, a strengthener of, rather than a substitute for a more unstudied awareness. A posture that sees theory as a tool for, not as a diversion from, nursing.

SOME GRANDER MISCONCEPTIONS AND A FEW GUIDES

Theory Development, Generally Speaking

DEVELOPMENT

At least three connotations are possible and in fairly current use for the word 'development'. A development might be regarded as happenings that chronicle change, whether or not the change is taken as progress toward a goal. To report development is, in another sense, to assess a pattern of change as to its pace or progress toward sophistication in adequacy, in scope, in amount, or in kind. In a third sense, to outline development is to describe or prescribe stages of, say, theory. These stages might be regarded as structural parts in interrelation, or they might be regarded as temporally related in their production. These ambiguities, now noted, are to be watched for; we have no intention of legislating them out of existence.

THEORY: SOME GROSS DISCRIMINATIONS AND A GUIDING PROPOSAL

When confusions of mere oversight are set aside, theory, however variously it is conceived, is distinguished (1) from doing or more physical processes; (2) from empirical reality as it is (in contrast with that reality as described, explained, predicted, or known); (3) from unarticulated awareness. Far less clear-cut is the going distinction, even in careless usage, between theory and (1) empirical generalization, (2) scientific laws, (3) hypotheses, (4) correlations, (5) speculations, (6) validated hypotheses, (7) operationalizations of abstract constructs or concepts, (8) conceptual constructs, (9) propositions relating theoretical entities or variables, and so on.

Still less clearly articulated habitually is what the component parts of theory are and how they are related, once some proposal or agreement is made as to the kind of being (or existence) theory has as opposed to that of non-theory.

Pertinent (and open) questions are these: (1) Is theory a set of concepts? (2) Is theory a set of hypotheses, laws, empirical generalizations, and so on? (3) Are all component parts of theory alike in kind? Are they all coordinate with one another? (For instance, in a hypotheticodeductive or axiomatic model of theory, the propositions or laws are seen as consequentially ordered rather than as merely coordinate.) (4) Are there levels or kinds of theory, whether in coordination or in some more intimate interrelation? Or is predictive theory the only theory properly so-called, and all other conceptualization either a preparation for such theory or an application of such theory? (5) Is it possible that there should be different theories covering the same area of phenomena and yet such that more than one of the theories is validated or good or true (even though they disagree one with the other in one, some, or many details)? (6) Is a theory good, valid, or true when it corresponds to reality? Or is some more sophisticated measure of a theory's propriety called for either because we cannot directly consult reality or because theoretical constructs necessarily go well beyond mere reflection of the empirical? (7) Is theory abstracted from reality by some process of induction or abduction? Does observation alone give rise to theory? Or is theory building more essentially inventive, however much validation depends on empirical observation? (8) Is any reporting of observation really theory-free? Is the empirical given unambiguously with respect to possible description? How does selection, expectation, theoretical or professional awareness affect what is noticed and the subsequent characterization of the noted?

In the context of these gross discriminations and open questions about theory, we offer a guiding proposal, which we have described in detail elsewhere [3–5]. To regard theory as a conceptual framework invented to some purpose has the virtue of allowing as subcases of theory so conceived other more traditional but more provincial notions of theory.

Distinguishing four kinds of theory – naming, correlating, predicting, and prescribing (or situation-producing) theory – helps emphasize two features about theory building. First of all, naming and correlating are not theory-innocent descriptions or observations; moreover, strengths, inadequacies, or biases in naming or correlating theories are reflected in predictive theory that takes them for granted, especially if the predictive theorist does not recognize the non-given status of naming and describing. Second, to see the possibility of a theory whose explicit purpose is to *produce* situations or reality of a given kind is a purposeful invitation. An invitation to what? To produce a guide to activity. But the invitation is to produce the guide not by a reliance on unarticulated or unsystematic or uninventive or untested "application" of predictive theory. Quite the contrary. The invitation is to produce a guide for activity by using extensions of already developed scientific techniques of invention, testing, and readjusting. (The current ecological crisis and vention, testing, and readjusting. (The current ecological crisis and the cry against technology are by-products resulting from the absence of such a theory. To remain at the level of thoughtless application or single-purpose engineering application of predictive theory is becoming patently unacceptable, even in the natural sciences, including the purest of physics.)

Each of the four levels of theory has distinctive components (as well as distinctive purposes). For example, naming theory has as components names or concepts seen either as merely coordinated or as more elaborately subgrouped in hierarchies. Naming is essentially tagging, so that taxonomy is a relation among names (often meant to reflect relations among things named). Names might also be called just concepts or constructs (or variables). However elaborate the concept, we would call it a tag or name if its purpose is to note a unity (as opposed purposefully to noting a correlation among unities). But correlating theory and predictive theory as opposed to naming theory have as components statements of relatedness. In correlating theory the relations are between conceived unities and so can be expressed in statements depicting states of affairs (or situations). In predictive theory the relations stated are *between* states of affairs. The question of whether something more elaborate than mere coordination exists among the components of correlating theory or predictive theory we leave an open question. But it is important to emphasize that for situation-producing theory the structure is essentially more complicated, since three distinctive kinds of components seem required (to fulfill the theory's purpose): statements of goal content; prescriptive statements; and listings of theories and other factors relevant to following prescriptions to produce situations that can be characterized by statement of goal content.

What makes a theory good, valid, or true; and how, for any theory, is the goodness discerned? We suggest that a good theory is a theory that fulfills its purpose. Once theory is seen as a conceptual invention to some purpose, this notion of good theory is plausible. Once it is realized that the proposal merely generalizes the notion of good theory most used in assessing predictive theory, the uneasiness about linking truth to purpose lessens.

APPROACH

Selective comment rather than exhaustive and antiseptic description about theory development is our intent. Moreover, precision suitable to the discussion immediately at hand rather than some pervasive and set level of conciseness is our policy here. These tactics of approach are a further overt challenge to the naive notions that there are absolute simples or beginning places; that an unbiased comment is possible; that total precision and explicitness is always the most effective mode of communication; and finally, that the floating but controlled ambiguity of common parlance is inappropriate in more learned discourse.

Some More Specific Reminders and Guides

THERAPY: FOUR DIMENSIONS OF MISCONCEPTION ABOUT THEORY

To speak of misconceptions seems to suggest criticism made in the light of an acknowledged right standard of what theory is – but to the contrary. Rather than contest about accepted usage (lexical definitions) or true conceptions (real definitions) of theory or anything else, we take a healthier orientation. Conceptions are proposals to be measured for their fruitfulness. From that orientation, to speak of misconceptions about theory is to speak of confusions, fixations, or even current usages that seem to be disruptive or inhibiting to progress in theory development.

Aristotle, in what now seems a quaint use of "cause," distinguishes material cause, formal cause, final cause, and efficient cause. The material cause of an entity is the stuff from which the entity is made. The formal cause is the defining structure or form of the thing. A thing's final cause is that for the sake of which the thing is or is brought into existence. The producing agent or agency is, finally, the thing's efficient cause. (This last sense of "cause" is probably closest to our more usual current usage.) One useful application of Aristotle's distinctions is for exploring a thing complex enough to have several interesting facets, for example, theory.

Theory's Matter or Stuff. What sort of entities or stuff make up theory? This is a basic question to ask about theory if we are self-consciously building theories. For how can one make a structure if he doesn't know what materials are the building blocks? In discussions of theory, expressions such as 'concepts', 'laws', 'empirical generalizations', 'operational definitions', 'scientific explanations', 'independent variable', 'causal implications', 'abducted generalizations', 'hypotheticodeductive system', and the like are freely and sometimes interchangeably used. Often, the expression 'theory' is identified with some one of the enumerated expressions. We have proposed as a useful notion of theory that to be theoretical is to be conceptual; that a theory is a conceptual entity, in particular, a conceptual framework invented to some purpose. What, then, is a concept? And how are concepts expressed?

Our tack is to propose a definition of concept in terms of the function a concept performs. A concept is a structuring device invented to enable the mind to regard disparate or distinguishable things as one or as united. Granting that a concept functions in this way, we can still ask what kind of "thing" a concept is. Is it a psychological event? A linguistic entity? A nonlinguistic entity such as a meaning? Or what? Asking these questions might be regarded as a quibbling were it not that discussion too often bogs down in confusion surrounding these various possibilities. Our proposal suggests a practical resolution of the question by an appeal to physical presentation – to what, roughly speaking, is the physical component of written language.

We begin by defining a *scratch presentation* ostensively (that is, by pointing to examples). We present some things that are scratch presentations and some that are not. Here is a scratch presentation:

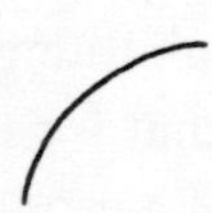

Here is another:

%

and another:

ible

and another:

pasquil

and still another:

concept

Among things that are not scratch presentations are the book you are reading, the chair on which you are sitting, an automobile, and Mount Rushmore.

When two scratch presentations have the same shape, we define them to be *like scratch presentations* (that is, to be scratch presentations that are alike in shape). For example, the scratch presentation

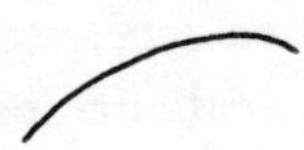

is like the scratch presentation

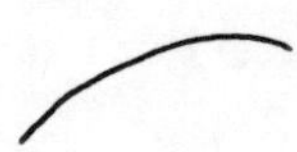

but unlike the scratch presentation

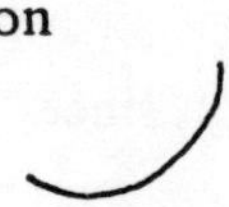

Likeness of scratch presentation can be ascertained without reference to meaning. Without knowing what meaning is being expressed or, indeed, if any meaning is being expressed, we can judge that:

bara

and:

bara

are like scratch presentations.

A *scratch pattern* (as opposed to a scratch *presentation*) is that in virtue of which two like scratch presentations are said to be like scratch presentations. A scratch *pattern* so defined is an entity different in kind from a scratch *presentation.* A scratch presentation is a physical entity, with a spatial, temporal location. Though what we call the *instances of a scratch pattern* are physical entities – specifically, scratch presentations – a scratch *pattern* is not a spatial, temporal object; a scratch pattern cannot be touched, smelled, destroyed, or located. A scratch pattern has, in logical jargon, the status of a universal in contrast to the status of a physical entity. In other jargon, a scratch pattern is a construct, the construct in virtue of which two like scratch presentations are said to be like presentations.

Our proposal for concepts can now be articulated. We propose that a *concept* is a scratch pattern to which meaning has been assigned. So a concept is not a physical entity, though only by means of physical entities have we access to concepts. Only in terms of our manipulation of physical entities – names, scratch *presentations* – are we able to use concepts. (A parallel discussion with respect to *sound* presentations could be given.) Still, we cannot touch a concept or even write one. For example, is

bara

a concept? Obviously not, since

bara

is a scratch presentation as opposed to a scratch pattern. So,

bara

cannot be a scratch pattern to which meaning has been assigned and thus cannot be a concept according to the proposed notion of concept.

Is

bara

an instance, however, of a concept, that is, an instance of a scratch pattern to which meaning has been assigned? In more common terminology, is the scratch presentation

bara

a word? (We propose that a word is an instance of a concept; so, in other terms, we propose that a word is an instance of a scratch pattern to which meaning has been assigned; that is, a word *is* a scratch *presentation* and is an *instance of* a concept [scratch pattern]). Mere inspection of the physical entities – within limits of tolerance of "sameness" – discloses whether or not the entities are like entities. Such "mere inspecting," however, does not reveal whether any meaning has been assigned or what specific meaning has been assigned to the corresponding scratch pattern. From mere looking we cannot tell whether the presentation is an instance of a concept. More particularly, though

ruler

and

ruler

or, say,

patient

and

patient

are (pairwise) like scratch presentations and so (for each pair) instances of the same scratch pattern, each member of a pair may be an instance of a different concept. Different meaning may be assigned to one and the same scratch pattern. A presentation as such is ambiguous with respect to the concept, if any, being expressed; for instance, a ruler may be a measure or a sovereign.

At the very least, our proposal regarding concepts brings to the surface two important features of concepts: first, that ambiguity is genuinely and inescapably present once language is used to express repeatable meaning; second, that if concepts are to function in expressing meaning as well as in being reusable and intersubjective, they must be entities of a less obvious kind than might be thought before reflection. (With respect to the complexity of our suggestions about concepts, see our remarks below about the complexity of our proposal about theory.)

How are concepts made if concepts are taken to be scratch patterns to which meaning has been assigned? Since a scratch pattern is an intangible nonsensible entity, how is meaning assigned to a concept (since a concept is, by our proposal, a scratch pattern to which meaning has been assigned)? And how is the assignment of meaning recorded or communicated? Our proposal suggests that the solution is by the manipulation of scratch presentations – in a word, via definition. Meaning is assigned to a scratch pattern by defining an instance of a scratch pattern (a scratch presentation, a word) and invoking the convention that all like scratch presentations are similarly defined. In general, to define a scratch presentation (a word, an expression) is to delimit that expression by saying that the expression denotes (refers to) exactly those things that can be denoted by the defining expression; or else, in the case of certain kinds of contextual definitions (including operational definitions), to say that the defined expression is true exactly in those cases in which the defining expression is true. Here we refrain from suggesting a useful grammar or logic of definition.

There are many ways of defining, and it is illuminating to classify definitions on the basis of structure of the defining expression. Noncontextual definitions are much used and are perhaps the simplest kind of definitions. Operational definitions are a well-known type of contextual definition, but there are other kinds of contextual definitions of comparable usefulness to the theory builder. Still, rather than articulating modes of definitions and ways of evaluating proposed definitions, our point here is to emphasize the kind of being or the ontological status of concepts and to suggest the manner in which such conceptual entities are related to the activity of defining.

Concepts can be distinguished from one another in various ways. One important classification of concepts has to do with the *referents* of a concept. Distinguish an instance of a concept (a word, a scratch presentation) from a referent of a concept: An instance of a concept is a linguistic entity – an instance of a scratch pattern to which meaning has been assigned; or, more briefly, a word. Since in the course of our discussion meaning has been assigned to the appropriate scratch pattern, we can now go on to say that

concept

is a word, that is, an instance of a concept. But the word

concept

is not a referent of the concept *concept.* In general, a referent of any concept is a "thing" – not necessarily a linguistic entity or even any other kind of physical entity – denotable by (named by, or pointed to by) a word expressing the concept (an instance of the concept). Thus, the concept *nurse,* the concept *patient,* the concept *patient-centered nursing* are referents of the concept *concept;* whereas each of the individual nurses in Massachusetts General Hospital are referents of the concept *nurse*, each of the individual patients referents of the concept *patient,* and each activity of patient-centered nursing a referent of the concept *patient-centered nursing*.

An individual nurse has a very different kind of being (different kind of ontological status) than the being of a concept *nurse*. And though concepts, as concepts, are like one another in the kind of being, or ontological status, they possess, still we might want to classify concepts on the basis of the kind of being their referents possess. For though all concepts have the same kind of being, the referents of various concepts may have various kinds of being. For instance, a referent of our proposed concept *concept* is not a physical being, but a referent of a concept *nurse* is usually intended to be a physical being, and any referent of our proposed concept *scratch presentation* is a physical being (a word). Scientific constructs are often concepts that have referents that are not physical entities, but

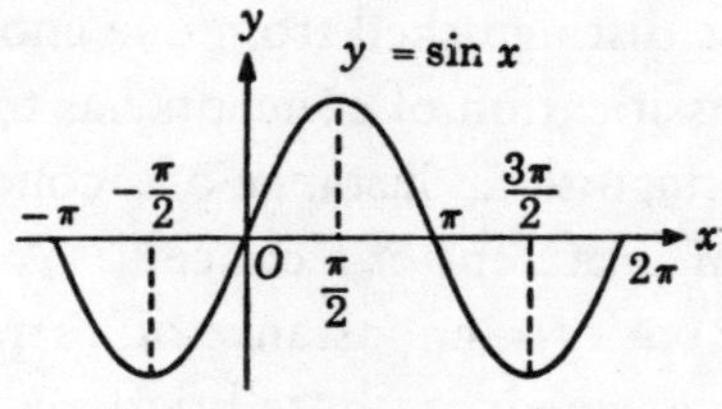

Figure. Graphic representation of symmetrical sine function such as that characteristic of a pendulum. (From Thomas, G. B., Jr. *Calculus and Analytic Geometry, Alternate Edition.* Reading, Mass.: Addison-Wesley, p. 179, Fig. 4-5 *a*, 1972.)

are such that by some indirect means we claim to link the referents of these constructs to empirical (physical) entities.

We call concepts whose referents are not physical entities *concepts by intellection* [6]. And concepts by intellection can be further distinguished. There are concepts by intellection that have pictures associated with them, for example, the concept *sine function* (see figure). For a graph reflects (pictures) some of the features possessed by a sine function (such as periodicity and symmetry), though a sine function is not a line or curve but rather is a (nonphysical) relationship (between numerical values). Other concepts by intellection have no picture associated with them; for example, a concept *fiscal policy* or a concept *Elizabethan age,* or perhaps a concept *concept.* Unmindful of the status of concepts by intellection, people often mistake the import of many scientific concepts: In a context of Freudianism one may wonder where his dream censor is, or speak of John's overactive id and Frank's underdeveloped superego. Such responses take a theoretical enterprise to be necessarily a word painting of what is the case and overlook the possibility that the conceptual enterprise that is theory may employ concepts by intellection.

Consider a further complication. Compare a concept *nurse* with a concept whose instance is

Few nurses earn more than doctors.

Unlike the first concept, whose instance is

nurse

the second concept (or its instance) can appropriately be said to be either true or false, most probably, true. It would be inappropriate, however, to say that the first concept, the concept *nurse*, is true or false. The concept *nurse* is not the sort of thing of which we could predicate truth or falsity. Concepts that may appropriately be said to be true or false are often called propositions, not concepts, though the entities have the ontological status of concepts. Ontologically speaking, propositions are concepts that can be true or false. Propositions can be regarded as formed from other concepts in one of two ways: A proposition is the result of joining nonpropositional concepts, as when the concept *nurse*, the concept *alleviate*, and the concept *pain* are joined to form the proposition that nurses alleviate pain. Or a proposition results from the joining of concepts that are already propositions. For example, a concept whose instance is

Nurses alleviate pain.

and a concept whose instance is

Nursing is still a much needed profession.

can be joined to form a concept whose instance is

If nurses alleviate pain, then nursing is still a much needed profession.

Traditional and modern logic suggests various ways that concepts can be related to produce propositions.

Our purpose here is to suggest that both the non propositional concept and the propositional concept are theoretical entities and that various kinds of collections of concepts, especially propositional concepts or propositions, exist. We can recognize as a collection of propositions a group created merely by enumerating propositions (by enumerating instances of these propositions), simply to create an arbitrary collection of propositions. But as human beings we do not as a rule engage in such purposeless collection, except when each individual researcher "adds" his one individual hypothesis (a name given to a proposition or its instance in virtue of the evidential status of that proposition).

The collection of propositions to which we attend are, by and large, groups of propositions that exhibit various kinds of interrelatedness. We may attend to a collection of propositions pertaining to a well-defined subject or subject-matter – say, the propositions describing the Elgin Marbles or propositions concerned with steel production in the United States. The propositions are related to one another in that each proposition in this collection deals with the Elgin Marbles; in that collection the propositions are related because each tells us something about United States steel production. But other sorts of relationships exist among propositions, in virtue of which the propositions are said to constitute a collection (or whole). For example, a deductive relationship could be a relationship by virtue of which we create a collection of propositions. The propositions in the group are such that one of them – call it the conclusion – is a logical consequence, in virtue of articulated rules of inference, of the group's remaining propositions, called the premises. More generally, a hypotheticodeductive theory might be regarded as a group or collection of propositions such that some of them, the axioms, give rise, by suitable rules of inference, to other of the propositions within the group.

The question of what is the stuff or material of theory is far from exhaustively answered here, but at least the outlines of an orientation to an answer, and a recognition of the question's propriety, should now be evident.

Theory's Form or Structure or Essential Characteristics. Misconceptions or unresolved confusions about the stuff of theory – what kind of entity it is as a whole, what kind of entities are its components, what kind of a thing a concept is – can give rise to many further confusions or inhibitions when one tries to build or use a theory. Misconceptions or confusions about the form, structure, or functional being of theory are also likely to give rise to difficulty in theory construction and use.

For example, what is it about a theory that makes the theory scientific? The possession of some given pattern or structure? Or is it rather the mode of invention and verification of the theory? The latter is at least plausibly the case. And once this possibility is seen, at least one objection is removed against the view that suggests that theory whose structure is less elaborate or else more complex than predictive theory could yet be scientific theory. For such theories could be validated empirically. How so? In terms of intersubjectively agreed-on conventions of confirmation. Does that answer still trouble you as a reader, as a hard-headed, "objective," researcher for Truth? If so, you must be clinging to a naive conception of objectivity as some sort of revealed or "seen" correspondence with the real. Break through this captivating though highly implausible myth that traps you as nurse-theoreticians. How? By seriously encountering the correspondence theory of truth. Subscribe so wholeheartedly to that view that you will be willing to state it clearly before the perplexed who don't grasp what you are about. When you say that a theory is true because it corresponds to the real, characterize the nature of the elements of theory, the nature of the elements of the real, and finally the nature of the correspondence. The proposition

Nightingale lies on the bed

corresponds to the real because 'Nightingale' denotes Nightingale, 'the bed' denotes the bed, and the relation expressed by the expression 'lies on' corresponds to the relation displayed by Nightingale on the bed. What could be clearer? Granted there are propositions for which such a correspondence account is plausible; otherwise, the hold the correspondence view of truth has on the mind would be difficult to explain. But can you make the account general? What will you do with

Most windows in the room are open.

The acceleration of bodies is a constant proportional to the impressed force on the bodies.

The kinetic energy of a gas is . . .

Once this naive notion of objectivity as correspondence is dispelled, the suggestion that the more complex type of theory –

situation-producing theory, for example – might get "objective" validation becomes the more plausible. Consider objectivity as the absence of mere subjectivity, as the possibility for intersubjective agreement. Then taking as the mode of validation intersubjective agreement within a professional community as opposed to throughout the wider community of *all* observers, however unskilled or untrained, is more easily appreciated as being no withdrawal from scientific objectivity realistically viewed. Isn't this approach functional even in the natural sciences, where the man in the street's lack of trained capacity does not bother the community of inquirers who can, thanks to their skill and training, come to agreement with respect to empirical criteria for validation? (An interesting example of a skill available perhaps to nurses [at least in obstetrics] but not even to, say, physicians, might be the hand-sensing of intensity or duration of labor contractions, perhaps not in every degree of difference but maybe as among practically important degrees of difference. Practicing nurses, as opposed to those more academically oriented, might present many other such examples.)

Here are some further related questions about theory. These questions seem to rise up persistently and cause disagreements, confusions, and distractions to more fruitful activities. (1) Is a theory as a theory different from a philosophy? (2) Is a situation-producing theory different from an application of a theory or from engineering based on pure theory? (3) Is practice theory different from a set of rules of practice? (4) Is theory that incorporates values and goals different from a statement of professional purpose? (5) Is theory – naming theory – different from a naming scheme or custom?

Besides the confusions to which these questions can give rise, they have in common also this not unrelated feature: They are better *not* answered by a simple yes or no. Rather than to legislate usage to give firm affirmative or negative answers, it is more to the practical point to see, for example, how a theory is like a philosophy and how unlike it; how a theory is like a set of rules and how unlike it.

Consider first the relation of a theory of nursing to a philosophy of nursing. Insofar as both are conceptual inventions, a theory and a philosophy do not differ. Furthermore, as possibly referring to some nonempirical entities, theory need not differ from philosophy; nor need the two differ when regarded as articulated guides to action. But unless we regard the conceptual invention as systematically exposed to empirical test, that invention is probably better not called theory, though the conceptual network might be called a philosophy, however dogmatically arrived at or held.

How is situation-producing theory like, how unlike, an applied theory or engineering based on pure theory? Considered merely as eventuating in the production of situations of a desired kind, situation-producing theory is like applied theory or engineering based on pure theory. Still they differ. Engineering (even as theory-based) is a relatively isolated and single-minded production of situations or commodities and *as engineering* attempts no explicit consideration of the total ramifications both of the means used and the ends produced. Similarly, situation-producing theory differs from the mere application of predictive theory where there is no documented – or at least no verbally communicable – procedure specified as to what constitutes the application. For education, duplication, justification, and especially revision, the explicit articulation of the guides to "application" are perhaps a very real practical contribution of situation-producing theory.

How is a set of rules of practice like and how unlike a situation-producing theory? As articulated guides to activity, the set of rules resembles a situation-producing theory. But insofar as the rules are regarded as specifying rigid and unalterable activities, the set of rules differs from a situation-producing theory. Moreover, in offering no explicit characterization of tendency or goal of the activities resulting from following the rules as guides, the set of rules is further unlike a situation-producing theory. Another difference is that the set of rules gives no clue as to how much they leave unspecified. Nor do the rules specify to what attention should be directed in resolving the practical ambiguities remaining, even given the rules. In situation-producing theory the survey list – with its enumeration of theories and other factors deemed relevant to production of activity according to the prescription so as to produce situations characterizable by the statement of goal content – serves this latter function.

In what ways does a situation-producing theory resemble a statement of professional purpose? In what ways does the theory differ from such a statement? If regarded as inviolable and not subject to compromise, a statement of professional purpose is essentially unlike a situation-producing theory, even though both include explicit characterization of goal. Moreover, insofar as the statement of professional purpose is taken as more noble or less scientific than other directors of activity, the statement differs essentially from a situation-producing theory. The two do not differ as containing an explicit statement of goal. Still, the goal content as specified in a situation-producing theory is necessarily viewed as temporarily specified and subject to revision just as much as any other part of the theory.

In addition, the goal content of the situation-producing theory is explicitly subject to considerations of feasibility, whatever compromise in ideal such subjugation might seem to require. Further, the goal content in a situation-producing theory is to be viewed as emerging from knowledge considerations, from professional experience, and from skills more than simply from personal value preferences. A situation-producing theory's statement of goal content may differ in yet another way from more pious and removed statements of professional purpose: The theory's statement of goal content is intended as a practical guide, supplementing the guides furnished by explicit prescriptions and a reminder list (survey list) for activity.

Finally, another more simple-minded question: When is a set of names best regarded as a naming theory? If the names are viewed as pre-given, objective, neutral tags for objective realities, the names are probably best not thought of as a theory. But when the names are viewed as consciously invented or selected for isolating atoms for attention, then to view some set of names as a naming theory is perhaps a practical move. Viewing the collection of names as alterable, as sources of difficulty, or as aids in further theoretical invention is to conceive them as a naming theory. Similarly, when the names function as convenient handles and so offer a kind of control – or at least serve as guide in activity – they can be practically viewed as a naming theory.

Theory's End or Purpose. Etymologically, the word 'theory' is linked to 'theorein', a Greek word meaning "to contemplate" or "look at," which in turn is linked to 'spectator' and 'theater'. To contemplate says Aristotle in his *Ethics*, speaking perhaps ironically, is man's most divine activity. Perhaps it is a religious impetus that makes us enshrine pure, contemplative knowing as so desirable. And yet, scientific method grows from Bacon's seventeenth-century revolutionary stance: Given that we have no direct illumination from reality, though we can have practical interaction with reality (experimentation), Bacon urged using "fruit," as he called it, as a clue to "light." How ironic, then, that proposing a theory with fruits, a theory whose aim is production of situations to a desired end is sometimes regarded as recommending an unscientific project! Historical accident together with a resulting overly narrow conception of theory – rather than some fixed dictate of theory as divinely conceived and laid up to be discovered – prevents the invention and use of theory to guide production of situations to a desired end. Even if the aim is merely to control nature, mere prediction as explanation leaves open the question of direction of desired control. And when control – or creation of social situations – and not just control of nature or production of commodities is at issue, then some guide beyond mere prediction is still more obviously needed for activity.

The enobling of theory viewed as solely explanatory or contemplative of truth stems in large part from the religious impulse. But in addition to this impulse, it is probably the desire of social scientists and would-be nurse-scientists to gain "scientific respect" through aping the procedures of theory suitable for the natural sciences that gives rise to the adulation of predictive theory and of theory as telling us what nature is (or how things stand). (See our remarks on p. 46 concerning understanding.)

Theory's Producers. Peplau [7] quotes Merton's conception of the interrelation of the various contributors to a discipline, with which she seems to agree:

The organization of science operates as a system of institutionalized vigilance, involving competitive cooperation. It affords both commitment and reward for finding where others have erred or have stopped before tracking down the implications of their results or have passed over in their work what is there to be seen by the fresh eye of another. In such a system, scientists are at the ready to pick apart and appraise each new claim to knowledge. This unending exchange of critical judgment, of praise and punishment, is developed in science to a degree that makes monitoring of children's behavior by their parents seem little more than child's play. Only after the originality and consequence of his work has been attested by significant others can the scientist feel reasonably confident about it. Deeply felt praise for work well done, moreover, exalts donor and recipient alike; it joins them both in symbolizing the common enterprise. That, in part, expresses the character of competitive cooperation in science [8].

In the same article by Peplau [7], the following is stated in an appended "Tool and Task Outline":

Competition is a tool of the juvenile era used in contesting for affection and/or status with others [p. 44].

Cooperation is [a?] to [sic] tool of the juvenile era which the child uses in maintaining his own position by adjusting and adapting to the wishes of others [p. 44].

The appendix goes on to state:

Collaboration is a tool in the preadolescent era which is a step forward from cooperation. Achievement is no longer a personal success in terms of "we." He moves from his desire to maintain his position in the group to derive satisfaction from group accomplishment [p. 44].

Granted that these quotations about competition, cooperation, and collaboration are taken from material prepared by graduate students, not by Peplau [see Note]. Still, the juxtaposed quotes are somewhat ironic – or, at the very least, suggestive. Especially with a professional group trying to be scientific, a less childish interplay among producers of theory would be perhaps more appropriate than the interplay suggested by Merton's words. That research tends to be done to gain a doctorate in a discipline outside of nursing may itself constitute a twofold invitation back to the more childish mode of interaction. Personal status rather than professional gain is surely part of the impetus supporting the expenditure of energy needed to endure the doctoral path. Moreover, taking the doctorate in a discipline outside nursing creates a demand and a desire to be distinctive, even as a nurse, and to make an idiosyncratic contribution to the more foreign discipline.

On the other hand, as suggested already, one of the obstacles to producing prescriptive theory (situation-producing theory) is the worry lest the activity be unscientific or unrespectable, either because it incorporates what seem merely personal biases or because it does not reveal further secrets of nature. An eccentric dependence on or overconcern about what other disciplines do or would say about what nurses do seems at times to make academic nurses do whatever will make them respectable in those foreign eyes, whether or not the activity adds an iota to nursing theory, research, practice, or education. By odd contrast, many nurses seem peculiarly insistent on defining the practical profession internally rather than by response to social demands or pressures of related practical disciplines [9].

In contrast to the desire to make idiosyncratic contributions, there seems to be among nurses a persistent demand to produce but *one* nursing theory – to get one respectable "body of knowledge" for nursing. From what does this desire stem? Perhaps it stems from overemulation of natural science as a discipline and from seeing natural science as offering a true description of nature; or from the fear that to admit there may be more than one nursing theory is to admit that such theories are just so many personal "philosophies" of nursing.

Delaying the production of nursing theory for the prior completion of all other non-nursing theories and all the lower level theories on which nursing is deemed to depend is another of those unrealistic postures nurses assume. The survey-list ingredient is included in the structure of a practice theory – among other reasons – to give explicit recognition to those areas about which awareness is wanted as well as to alert users to the need for creating knowledge in some of these areas. Practical awareness is a likely source of identification of these areas (as may be theoretical and academic broadness and sophistication). That is, one of the jobs of the would-be producers of nursing theory would be to spell out areas for which theory from other disciplines is wanted and perhaps also to provide the impetus in those disciplines for getting those theories produced.

A more realistic conception of who are the theory experts for nursing is perhaps also needed. At the First Nursing Theory

Conference (Kansas, 1969) pride was expressed [10] because the participants were not just deans but included two "Executive Directors of Nursing Services." There were some 40 participants. Is the ratio of 1 to about 20 a suitable measure of the role the practitioner should play in setting priorities, furnishing realistic background, and supplying feasibility hunches? Surely, an appropriate way of suitably emulating the scientific community includes consulting of the empirical. The empirical reality most relevant to nursing theory may well be that reality available to the practicing nurse.

Though group production of theory is not much discussed, synthesis in another sense is considered an important notion for nursing theory [11]. But why not regard the theoretical activity of synthesizing as focusing or extending concepts or theories from other disciplines so as to show their link to prescription and goal in nursing? To regard synthesis in this way may be more fruitful than to regard synthesis as some mystical gluing – a gluing done by a nurse equipped with information from a variety of disciplines and yielding a whole true picture. Nursing eclecticism is surely suitable to some purpose and priority!

Going On: Some Next Steps

Some of the reminders we are assembling here are selected by us at least partially in reaction, direct or indirect, to our reading of the *Proceedings* of the three Kansas theory conferences [12]. Those conferences might, in a sense, be expected to exhibit some of the more enlightened awareness about theory and theory activity in nursing. Moreover, misconceptions, confusions, dilations, and distractions evidenced there are probably representative of the larger nursing-theory community, since leaders were asked to the Kansas conferences. Our present suggestions for going on take off from, so to speak, and go beyond, the notion of assembling in conference *academic* leaders for *talk* about theory development. Without contriving overly, we can suggest – corresponding to each of the theory dimensions we distinguished for purposes of talking about misconceptions – a next step or two.

The Stuff or Grammar of Theory. Within most nursing curricula, tradition already supports a course on concepts in nursing. Strengthen that tradition. Instead of a course that merely explores more or less vigorously some basic notions of the profession of nursing, include within every nursing curriculum, however basic, a course on training nurses in the skill of conceptualization. Such a course aims to make conceptualization a *usable tool* for nursing. To analyze, criticize, and appreciate – rather than just passively to receive – materials used in the more traditional concepts course might still be appropriate. But now, instead of being just a source of information, these materials would be used to provide a field for exercising the skills acquired in a course, in which conceptualization is taught as a tool. The materials used for this latter purpose could include both historical matter from nursing, textbooks on nursing concepts, and current nursing research literature.

It seems important that this course or training in conceptualization be available long before the doctorate or master's level of training and available to all nurses – those destined for direct practice and administration, as well as for those aiming at academic careers in nursing or more research-centered nursing activity. Practitioners, as informed consumers and perhaps eventually as skilled demanders of research, need competence in and respect for conceptualization. Our contention is that even for direct practitioners and administrators, conceptualization skill, with its accompanying strengthening of communication and articulation, is a support of "thoughtful" nursing practice. Elsewhere [13] we have discussed how we think a more substantial use of conceptual approach could offer economies as well as improvements in nursing education.

The Function, Form, or Structure of Theory. Review of the literature is an established practice. We suggest that the reviews be enlarged in scope. Review existing nursing theories for their contents, but include in the survey an assessment and comparison of the structural features of these theories. Such reviews could serve both to train nurses in alertness to structural features of theory and to make them more aware of the state of current and past contributions in nursing literature. Moreover, we would suggest that this practice of careful review of the literature become a habit at each state of nursing education, however basic. The practice of review of the literature seems now too often reserved as a *devoir* or duty required to supply "Section I" of a publishable paper or an acceptable dissertation – an exercise to preface the report of "my" more idiosyncratic study. In nursing research there is an understandable emphasis on the need for originality and laissez-faire freedom. But needed now in such circles is a counterbalancing emphasis on joint endeavor and on appreciation of what has been done already by others, or what is now being done by others.

Furthermore – and in this same spirit – research for a practice discipline requires a peculiar kind of assessment of findings. The findings should be assessed as to their feasibility for practice. Nurses in actual service might be a source of fruitful contribution to such assessment. Assessing in this mode would be invaluable to potential researchers and to student nurses. Such assessment would alert researcher and nurse to two strands: (1) to the possibility of conceptual contributions to nursing practice and (2) to the factors beyond methodological propriety as defined by social or natural sciences, but factors that nonetheless are relevant to doing or using nursing research or to building nursing theory. That in-service education be used to make use of experienced personnel's assessments of feasibility is perhaps not an inappropriate move, especially if some avenue of communication could be arranged so as to make the output of such assessments available to students, neophyte nurses, or academic or research nurses.

The Purpose or End of Theory. Perhaps theory and research-oriented nurses should devote some of their energies to creating in the practice community expectations from theory and research. Should not the market be cultivated for research, the commodity prized – or at least bought at so great a cost in energy and dollars – by one segment of nursing, the group called, perhaps suitably, nursing leaders? In nursing education, however basic, perhaps what must be cultivated and taught is the *use* of research and theory. That capacity is surely as important for a practice discipline as the skills for the production of research and theory. The suggestions given about courses in the skill of conceptualization and developing the habit of literature review are steps in developing a capacity to use research and theory.

Should not energies be directed to showing specifically how

theory and research make tangible practical differences in nursing. Or – more honestly – we need to articulate in what ways fruits from theory and research have fallen short of expectation (see "What Difference Does It Make?"). And perhaps service personnel, and not just head nurse or nursing directors, should begin to be nonpatronizingly consulted by graduate students in nursing as well as by theorists and researchers for some advice on problems and priorities for guiding nursing investigations. These latter interplays might serve two functions: supplying insights on where energies should be directed first or with greatest emphasis; and beginning at least to cultivate the notion among practitioners as well as researchers that there is and ought to be a more realistic relation between the interests and preocuppations of the two. As soon as the consultation is nonpatronizing, then the inquirers might also cultivate a more direct and authentic communication with practitioners, so that in joint sessions, mutual contempts might be handled verbally and exploited for the good of nursing rather than submerged politely when together and then, once conferring is done, used in mutual deprecation.

Theory's Producers. Has not the moment for concentrating on individual inquiry and individual interests passed? Perhaps a conference should be arranged to deal explicitly with setting up current priorities for areas of research and theory building for nursing. The conference might try to assess who best could do what needs to be done for nursing, whether within or outside nursing, and might concentrate also on commissioning the work deemed needed. Perhaps the time for preoccupation with precisely what theory is and what structure it should have is passed – or has not yet arrived. Isn't nursing ready for a more aggressive use of its new tools? Here is one way to begin to mobilize nursing's great manpower resources to this end: Use students much more extensively than now in a coordinated attempt to produce, for example, baseline data, and to replicate or use already existing study designs to collect massive enough data to give more than trivial sample populations. Providing students with research or theory activity that is not mere course busywork, that is not just idiosyncratic "my study" excursions into attempts at originality, might produce some substantial evidence or data for nursing.

This move might begin to cultivate a habit of seeing inquiry as a nonacademic exercise. To do such inquiry as a group endeavor might also have a beneficial effect on students as individuals. Group research might diminish traumas and the subsequent hate directed toward theory and research by at least some students when they are required to go through the motions of producing an acceptable piece of "independent research." With the attempt to incorporate research attitudes at more and more basic levels of nursing, the move to make the activity both "do-able" and productive becomes more important than ever. Moreover, to support and encourage students in such activities supplies a ready source of the currently much demanded "relevance." And is there any reason why in-service education could not similarly supply a coordinating source for research done by practitioners? (More than once we have heard practitioners remark enviously, and even with a dash of contempt, that with the time at the disposal of those who do nursing studies, they, the service nurses, could do something worth doing!)

MORE SPECIFIC DIFFERENCES

Some "differences" or confusions concerning theory for nursing arise more specifically in reactions to the mode of presenting or to the content of our proposals about theory. It seems to us, however, that others of the difficulties are more specifically related to the special fact of *nurses* now attempting to integrate theory and research into a profession that historically qua profession has habitually taken neither the theoretical stance nor the research stance.

We have proposed that theory be looked on not monolithically but as having four distinctive levels (or as being of four structural kinds, or as having four possible purposes or tasks). The levels we distinguished we picture thus:

Level I Factor-isolating theories (naming theories)
Level II Factor-relating theories (descriptive theories or depicting theories)
Level III Situation-relating theories
A. Predictive theories (time or direction relations of situations)

B. Promoting or inhibiting theories (speed, intensity, or scope of situations)

Level IV Situation-producing theories (prescriptive theories)

The levels are named here so as to make somewhat clearer how one level is related to another. At level I conceptualizations are made to isolate factors; then at level II the isolated factors conceived as related are used to describe situations. The next level, the third, conceptualizes relations as between situations described. Finally, the fourth level conceptualizes modes of producing situations of a specified kind.

Leave aside the question of whether it is not just soft-soaping or patronizing for us to propose that nursing theory is fourth-level theory and more structurally sophisticated than, say, physics conceived as a predictive theory. Leave aside, too, the question of whether it is ridiculous to grace with the name of theory the lowly activity of naming, even if naming is an inventing of a conceptual framework to some purpose. Still, our proposal that theory – a conceptual framework invented to some purpose – is fruitfully regarded as having levels before and after the predictive level (situation-relating theory) raises these questions: Which level is for the sake of which other level? Level IV is for the sake of what, if each preceding level is for the sake of the next level? And level I comes from what?

Further, is the order of production of the levels of theory the same as the order of enumerations – 1,2,3,4? Is the production of theory a linear development from factor-isolating to situation-producing theory? Is nursing theory exclusively fourth-level theory? To what extent does nursing theory include – rather than just depend on – other levels of theory?

We suggest that the whole enterprise of theorizing is best viewed as aimed at using conceptualization to make desirable differences in reality. We do not see theorizing as a contemplative affair, however much contemplation must be used as a tool in producing theory. Nor do we regard the intellectual comfort of having an "explanation" as a satisfying aim of the theorizing enterprise, however much aesthetic or speculative pleasure comes from attaining certain theoretical stances. In other words, we do not find theorizing a self-justifying enterprise.

We bother to isolate factors that we might relate them. We bother to relate factors and thereby describe situations so that we may begin to conceptualize relations as among those described situations. But why do we bother to "understand" or theorize about predictions, promotions, and inhibitions with respect to situations (states of affairs)?

Our suggestion is that we so conceptualize in order to allow ourselves to conceptualize further – but to the end now of actually bringing about, producing in practice or reality, situations to the specification of the practitioner or realist using the fourth-level theory. So, fourth-level theory is specifically and obviously not meant just to prepare some further possibility for theory (nor research meant for the sake of more research). Probably, it is a conscious or unconscious religious or thoughtlessly reverent attitude toward "pure thought" or "absolute truth" – a need for consolation because of a failure to produce any useful theory – that allows us self-righteously to hold to the notion that producing theory for the sake of producing theory is an enterprise of worth.

On what does first-level theory depend? Our proposal is that factor-isolating (naming) theory depends on practice, or activity in the "real," though of course some naming theories may depend on other, already existing, naming theories. These views about first-level and fourth-level theory lead us to propose that theory begins and ends in practice. Another way to put the matter is to say that theory, thetic activity, presupposes the nonthetic – awareness through modes other than merely the articulately conceptual.

From a structural point of view, fourth-level theory presupposes third-level theory; third-level theory presupposes second-level theory, and so forth. But from the point of view of production, a less orderly and less linear relationship is likely to hold. Third-level theory may have been consciously produced. But first- and second-level theory have probably been done only almost athetically, often with no consciousness that we are conceptualizing or taking over a ready-made conceptualization. Even after explicit beginnings of theory at the various levels, development may proceed erratically. Work on predictive theory may bring us to return to factor-isolating or merely descriptive theory; attempts to do fourth-level theory may well show us the need for as yet undeveloped predictive theories, and so on.

We have proposed that nursing theory is or should be a fourth-level theory. But once the interrelationship of levels is understood, it begins to be somewhat clearer how nursing theory would depend on other levels of theory. Specifically, we have proposed that the ingredients of nursing theory as a situation-producing theory would comprise (1) goal content, (2) prescriptions, and (3) a survey list. The survey list is, in a sense, the explicit enumeration of those theories at other levels and from other disciplines on which the production of desired nursing situations is conceived to depend, even though the conception is not as yet explicit as to what that dependence exactly is.

What does our proposal as to the ingredients or structure of situation-producing theory reflect? The recognition that to express a theory that could be functional in directing activity towards the production of reality to a desired end requires something more than just a collection of propositions, even if deductively related and regardless of whether or not they are causal (see pp. 59–60). More specifically, we want to emphasize that practice theory – as theory that could guide activity – needs to be more than a description of the real world, even if the description includes predictions.

Our proposal suggests that goal content (value orientation) needs to be given theoretical status. In a theory for activity, bias or purpose must be rendered explicit within the theory. Moreover, the goal content, like any other part of a theory, should be regarded as subject to change. But subject to change in the light of what? In the light of the goal content's interrelation with other parts of the theory; or in light of the relation of the theory as a whole to practical empirical reality; or in light of the theory as a whole to the aim of the proposing theoretician or of the practitioner who is using it. To put the matter in other words, to emphasize that even goal content has theoretical status and is subject to change suggests that (1) more than one nursing theory might be proposed; that (2) several nursing theories might usefully coexist (since any change in content or even in degree of specificity with any ingredient would constitute, in a sense, a change in theory); and that (3) values as they function in nursing are something more than mere personal values of the individual practitioner.

To make the survey list a part of the structure of situation-producing theory, in addition to the ingredients of goal content and prescriptions, is to incorporate certain recognitions explicitly into the theory's structure: (1) the recognition that there are matters relevant to goal and prescription not, or not yet, explicitly incorporated into the theory; (2) the recognition that the detail of doing or activity in the real is essentially inexhaustible in conception; and (3) the recognition that theory production is essentially ongoing and never finished.

We have proposed that the survey list be organized to reflect an activity's six aspects that might be particularly relevant to take into account in doing or in conceiving for doing. An aspect is a viewpoint on, rather than an integral part of, a whole. The six aspects we suggest are a generalization in a sense of Aristotle's fourfold causal analysis of reality. We have proposed that the survey list be organized along dimensions that parallel these six noteworthy aspects of reality: agency, patiency, framework (context or matrix), terminus, procedure, and dynamics. These aspects correspond to these questions:

Agency: Who or what performs the activity?
Patiency: Who or what is the recipient of the activity?
Framework: In what context is the activity performed?
Terminus: What is the end point of the activity?
Procedure: What is the guiding procedure, technique, or protocol of the activity?
Dynamics: What is the energy source for the activity?

We have suggested this scheme, which is more elaborate than ends, means, context, and doer, for a variety of reasons. One is to call nursing theorists' attention to elements in nursing beyond the mere nurse-patient dyad. Moreover, we wished to provoke a generalization from the traditional points of focus – nurse as agent, patient as patient or recipient – in order to encourage a more open, reflective, and innovative attitude, at least at the theoretical level, toward nursing realities or the possibilities for analyzing these realities or producing them. We feel it especially important to call attention to the need for theory's taking account of dynamics, the energy source of professional activity. Why? To focus attention, for example, on what besides service orientation can, is, or ought to be depended on as a power source for activity realizing the nursing goal [14].

We coined the name *situation-producing theory* for the fourth level of theory rather than use *normative theory* or *prescriptive theory*. Why? To emphasize the aim rather than just the structure or nature of such theory. As a matter of fact, we named each of the levels according to the aim or end point of that level of theory, though, of course, we suggest, too, that as the aim or purpose of the conceptualization changes, the structure needs to change in order that the theory achieve its purpose. But the term *situation-producing theory* has produced some difficulties. What do we mean by *situation*? And are we claiming that situations (the real) produce the theory? Some persons have interpreted our emphasis on the interesting and fruitful relation between the literally dumb, that is, unarticulated, awareness of the doer and what needs to be articulated to help come to a viable practice theory to mean that we are proposing that situations produce the theory [15]. And oddly enough, the contrary assumption has been made also [16].

Our intent is to emphasize that situations are to be produced, not just described. That is, situations are to be brought about, effected, made to happen. To call fourth-level theory situation-*producing* emphasizes what? That the purpose of such theory is to bring about desired differences in reality, not just by controlling reality or predicting it, but by shaping or producing reality to fit our specifications. To make this proposal is not to make the naive claim that "wishing makes things so." Far from it! Instead, we suggest that one of the strongest tools available for getting what we wish is *conceptual* awareness (a theory) of (1) more nearly what we wish (goal content); (2) what activity we should do to produce such a wished-for happening (prescription); and (3) what should be kept in mind in trying to produce the desired end (survey list).

To call fourth-level theory a situation-*producing* theory underscores that what we do as practitioners does in fact shape reality, for good or for ill, either to our wish or not. To be a professional or practitioner necessarily involves acting in the light of aim (call it bias, if you wish). To be a professional is – like it or not – to inflict our aims, especially our professional ones, on the clientele served. Such a realization should help make the practitioner the more eager to use whatever tools, including theory, that might be at his disposal. Why? To make more certain what those aims are and whether or not he is following the ones he thinks he is or would like to think he is following.

So much for production or producing. Now what is a situation? By situation, we do not mean a predicament or fix or a problem. Perhaps we should have anticipated the confusion. But philosophically, a situation is spoken about as a state of affairs. We chose the word to distinguish such states of affairs from mere isolated factors that might be singled out as ingredients in states of affairs. A proposition expresses a state of affairs. But a concept expressed by a noun (or the grammatical equivalent) expresses a factor, rather than a complex of factors united to produce a whole, which whole cannot exhaustively be characterized by the factors cited. A proposition expresses a state of affairs; and if the state of affairs exists, then the existence of the state of affairs is what is often called a fact.

We have been looking at the difficulties that seem to stem from the very content or mode of presenting our theory of theories. There are other difficulties that seem to stem more specifically from our attempts to deal with *nursing* theory as situation-producing theory and to direct our remarks to an audience of *nurses.* We have encountered a variety of nursing reactions to our notions on theory. The reactions are not necessarily consistent with one another. The sampling we give here is random and nonexhaustive. The description of the reactions is unabashedly our viewpoint on the nature and possible source of the reactions.

Some of the typically nursing reactions to our notions of theory stem, we think, from intellectual confusions or fixations. The apprenticeship mentality still fairly rampant in nursing (and other health disciplines) brings with it two convictions. First, professional judgment or "mystique" is essentially irreducible to conceptualization, hence why bother trying to theorize? Second, a conviction that professional education beyond basic sciences should be a kind of supervising carried on to point out apprentices' errors and to allow the apprentices to watch the great practitioner perform. The notion of an adequate telling or instructing and then relatively unsupervised doing is less than universally popular. There is more a preoccupation with sinlessness and freedom from dangerous consequences than with a sense of craftsmanship and independent accomplishment. In such an apprentice-type education, articulated theory has little place.

Where attempts are made by nurses to theorize, some odd ambivalences are sometimes manifested. On the one hand, theory is regarded as some magnificent achievement. Then nurses ask, "How can lowly nurses produce it?" Or, "How could it be possible that nursing does have (or has had) any theory that might be called a theory of nursing?" Conversely, as soon as theory is explicated as something attainable, even by a practitioner, the question arises in nurses as to whether something so attainable is worth aspiring to, or whether so practical a tool as situation-producing theory is not beneath the dignity of a nursing elite aspiring to make nursing a learned discipline.

Moreover, where we at times very purposefully emphasize an ambiguity and try to maintain that ambiguity, not infrequently the nurses, especially scientifically oriented nurses, try to push us to a neat resolution of the unsettling ambiguity [17]. For example, to talk in terms of goal, prescription, and survey list and to talk of the aspects of agent, patient, framework, terminus, procedure, and dynamics – is that to talk of theory structure, or of reality structure, or of nursing practice structure? We would answer, "Not one or the other of these but purposely all three." One of the virtues of our proposals about theory is that they are similarly useful as proposals for what should be the knowledge process appropriate to a nurse even as a practitioner and not just as a producer of theory.

Nursing reactions to our proposal of goal content as an ingredient of nursing theory include these two: On the one hand, there is a reticence to treat the nursing goal merely as a theoretical entity, perhaps because nurses are imbued with the notion of nursing as a commitment to service – a matter of heart and value, not just of head. On the other hand, we have encountered a certain unwillingness to admit that nursing as a profession has a bias and that in being a profession, nursing necessarily inflicts its values (bias) on those whom it serves. Our talk about situation-producing theory makes nurses uneasy because they do not want knowingly to manipulate or exploit people. Our discussion of the dynamics of nursing and our insistence that unmentionables should be mentioned offend nurses by reminding them that love and service motivation are not their only sources of motion. Finally, our reminder that a broader conceptual outlook suggests that perhaps patient-centered nursing, somewhat as task-centered nursing, is a mistake or, at least, a nonfruitful or even somewhat dishonest aim seems to some to take away the very birthright of nurses or point of nursing. Moreover, our richer conception of theory might allow some current practice to be called nursing, a consequence described by a fervent research-oriented academic nurse as "shocking."

WHAT DIFFERENCE DOES IT MAKE?

Theory and Research for Nursing: Jibe and Probe

Some find our view of theory difficult; some, nurses among them, suggest that it is too complex for nurses. Bertrand Russell's [18] observation is perhaps to the point.

> I will only beg the reader not to make up his mind against the view [Russell's theory of denotation] – as he might be tempted to do, on account of its apparently excessive complication – until he has attempted to construct a theory of his own on the subject of denotation. This attempt, I believe, will convince him that, whatever the true theory may be, it can not have such a simplicity as one might have expected beforehand.

But rejection because of complexity is not the only problem. Still, new outlooks can be taken in, in the invidious sense, as slogans and, thus transformed into shibboleths, are done in. New ideas are often misunderstood or distorted. How easy is it to generalize falsely from the striking example, to fix obstinately on some isolated aspect of a new thought; or without penetrating to intent, to give blind lip service because the perspectives are new. Such acceptance is another mode of rejecting a theory.

Acceptance or rejection of any proposed theory is a minor matter compared to the question of the nursing worth of the theoretical enterprise itself. Let us hurl at the theoretical enterprise the skeptical jibe, "What difference does it make?" The skeptical stance has its own integrity. So let us not confuse a sincere skeptic with an ill-tempered naysayer who wails and deprecates only to stultify activity or to protect the status quo. But as sincere skeptics, we cannot rest with the general indictment, "What difference does it make?" As soon as we assume the posture of sincere skeptic, the "logic" of the stance demands that our cutting jibe become a more discerning probe.

What is this "it" about which we are so exercised when we say, "What difference does it make?" The awareness of what theory is, or might be? The awareness of what *nursing theory* should be, structurally speaking? The awareness of *a particular nursing theory* with these structural features? Nor is specification of the "it" sufficient to render the jibe a probe. In whichever of these ways the "it" is taken, for that "it" one can still ask, *To whom does "it" makes a difference – for what?* To the nurse-theoretician, with her concern about the intended use of theory or about the intended users of theory? To the nurse-researchers, perhaps, concerned about research's role in theory development or the role of practice demands in their relation to both theory and research, or about non-nursing contributions to nursing? Or is the challenge of significance made by the nurse-educator who asks, What difference does the "it" imply for *mode, content,* and *economy* of instruction? Or perhaps the question is asked by the nurse-practitioner with respect to the level of care and the persistence of quality care. Or the nurse-practitioner, troubled by the inflexibility (or excessive flexibility) of the practitioner in the light of changing realities, or concerned with the expense of quality care, may demand what ramifications are to be found for the problem if the "it" is accepted. Or does the practitioner question the "it" for the implications concerning nurses' capacity to have professional identity, given both the pressing demands of reality and the demands of other non-nurse professionals?

For each of the probing questions, it is possible to suggest how the "it" could make a difference to the person in question for the task at hand. And it is possible to suggest how we could test whether or not the difference anticipated by reflection materialized in experience. Such a project is too detailed for our intent here. But in response to and in the spirit of the jibing skeptic we say: Unless "it" makes a difference for you in your aim, stop doing it. Fundamental to the view of practice theory we put forth is that practice theory is nothing but a tool or device to bring about a desired end, a tool which, ontologically speaking, is a conceptual entity but nonetheless is a tool. That nurses should engage in nursing theorizing for the sake of theorizing is foreign to our view of practice theory. That nurses should spend their time in developing nursing theory or engaging in nursing research simply for the intrinsic worth of these activities is in the light of our view of theory and research a waste of nursing energy.

There is much talk nowadays about developing nursing theory. But developing theory means what? To hold conferences, to read papers, to speculate, to put in time – all of this while we leave practice untouched? The old guard, because it is the old guard, take the stance of stultifying skepticism toward the whole enterprise of theory for nurses. The Young Turks take a stand for "nursing theory," hold symposia, and "feel" the call of a bright future. But the truth of the matter is that nursing practice is relatively untouched by either side, nor has nursing research had any considerable impact on nursing practice. Invited to speak in a symposium concerned with nursing research, we were given as title of our talk, "Nursing Research Having Payoff for Nursing Practice." In not being followed by a question mark, the title is a tip-off. At best, the research is done and *then* examined to determine how it might have payoff for practice. And isn't *that* a reasonable thing to do? We theorize, we research, and then we see how the findings can be implemented in practice. *In a sense, nothing could be more unreasonable.* The procedure puts the cart before the horse and divorces nursing practice (doing) from nursing thinking (theorizing and researching).

Why bother to theorize and to research? Our contention is that nursing practice is the alpha and omega of nursing theorizing and nursing research. The impetus for nursing theorizing and researching must arise from practice, since nursing is a practice. To deny that the theoretical stance, that is, conceptualization, makes a desirable difference for practice is to leave practice to the rule of rigid habit or of blind impulse. We are not claiming that most of, or even a goodly proportion of, the nursing theorizing going on today arises from practice and alters practice for the better. But we do affirm that nursing theory has this potential and that *without this payoff there is no justification for the enterprise of nursing theorizing.*

Insofar as the practitioner brings existing practice to conceptual awareness, she is theorizing. The nurse who, immersed in the reality of doing, records conceptually the awareness got in practice engages in rudimentary theorizing. The nurse as theorist or as researcher must exploit, that is, midwife, the nurse as practitioner for that awareness of nursing obtainable only by doing. Undoubtedly it is unrealistic to suppose that one and the same person will simultaneously have as goals giving service, producing theory for the consumption of others, and engaging in explicit research. More realistically, in practice disciplines there is a triad of "speculators": the practitioner, the theory builder, and the theory tester or researcher [19].

Theory can arise from practice if, for example, the theorizer exploits the awareness of the practitioner as to what constitutes the present practice, what are the unmet demands, what are the constant obstacles that thwart the practitioner. If theory and research are to be relevant to practice, they must be directed to the problems of nursing as now practiced. To bring about here and now a more effective guide for nursing activity than we now possess, the task of the theorizer and the researcher is to forge a tool: for the theorizer, a conceptual framework; for the researcher, a methodology sufficient to yield not merely significance according to norms of some social science but a significance in the light of nursing practice. Our suggestions as to the structure of practice theory and our remarks on the function of research were guided with that end in view.

Generalizing the Technique of Jibe-Probe: The Spirit of the Enterprise

Rather than being embarrassed by the skeptical jibe, "What difference does it make?" we welcome it as directed toward our theory of theories. In fact, we urge the general adoption of the constructively skeptical stance. Embrace the jibe, "What difference does it make?" but transform it into a probe. The jibe hurled from outside the relevant ranks is often intended as a war cry preceding attempts to change or cut down the "it" in question. Within the ranks, such a jibe is too often a defensive and protective reaction that reflects a certain joy or strength in the union against the common enemy who hurls the criticism.

We suggest a more self-conscious, self-initiating offensive use of the jibe-probe technique as a constructively self-critical tool within the ranks. Transform the jibe into a probe: specify the "it"; articulate to whom the "it" makes a difference for what. Then, with these specifications in mind, explore the enterprise under question. Such a habit of probing prevents too easy acceptance of fashionable intellectual fads which, though perhaps exciting, serve our purpose little. And too, such a transformed jibe is a constructive move of inquiry that requires our "discriminating the question." Such a move to distinction-making tends to throw an area into a new light and to bring into focus aspects and dimensions not always visible.

Let the question, "What difference does it make?" be uttered not as a cry of despair because some task looks overwhelming or looks to be of little or no significance in proportion to the outlay of time, energy, and funds. Let the question function not as a cry of mere "againstness" or withdrawal but as an honest guide to a positive program of self-scrutiny. To allow yourself to ask, "What difference does it make?" is not necessarily to require discarding the "it" that is. The question needs to be asked in the spirit of inquiry rather than in a spirit of despair or defense. To see "What difference does it make?" as a version of the question of significance suggests that the jibe-probe method is really the importing of the spirit or medium of true research into nursing itself; *by this move, the research spirit is integrated into the whole of nursing and does not constitute a mere diversion for the nursing elite.* For nursing to use the jibe-probe technique requires – besides a spirit of inquiry – self-esteem, the capacity to detect, admit, and survive error, strength, and commitment to nursing rather than to extraneous outside forces.

There is no need to restrict the question, "What difference does it make?" to theory or research in nursing. The same question might properly be raised to probe, say, the commitment to baccalaureate education in nursing or to associate degree programs in nursing. Furthermore, the jibe-probe technique need not restrict itself to being guided merely by the question, "What difference does it make?" Jibes are often hurled in other relatively harsh terms. Here are some forms such jibes might take:

> Why should nurses bother with theory? How can they? Why can't a nurse tend to her basically more practical task?
>
> What staff nurses would partake of continuing education were it not a paid release from real nursing responsibility or drudgery?
>
> Why do nurses in service have such contempt both for the endeavors and output of nursing research, especially as reported prettily to them in sessions of in-service education where researchers "share" findings for the enlightenment of the mere practitioner?

These jibes are not gentle, but they may be kind to nursing. To soften the question is not necessarily merciful. But to redirect the energy of taunt, derision, or assault (or the reactions to them) into more usefully thoughtful probes is the more constructive and hence ultimately the more genuinely protective move for nursing. For example, the theory jibe could become more probing when translated into the more discerning question:

> In what sense, if any, should every nurse be a theoretician? Distinguish these modes of encounter with theory:
>
> a. Producers of theory
> b. Conscious users of theory
> c. Unconscious users of theory
> d. Critic of theory
> e. Expositor of theory

f. Educator of others in the light of theory, where others can be:

   LPN
   RN of diploma school
   RN of college program
   RN of associate degree program
   RN in higher education, postgraduate
   MD
   the public

GOING ON: A NEW OPENNESS?

The Spirit of Knowledge Versus the Body of Knowledge for Nursing: The New Posture

In the hands of a person determined to build rather than to destroy, the skeptical stance can be transformed into a constructive – that is, helpful – probing. And more important to nursing than the criticism itself is the constructive critical spirit. This spirit is unwilling to rest in idle vacuities; this spirit actively works to create the endeavor realizing the nursing aim. So conceived, the critical spirit *is* the theoretic stance, in our sense of theory.

Many and frequent have been the demands for a "body of knowledge" for nursing. *Would the cultivation of a spirit of knowledge for nursing be more fruitful than the barren search for a "body of knowledge" specific to nursing? Emphasis on techniques of ongoing inquiry and openness of mind to new ways and possibilities might be healthier than attempts to establish new dogmas or rigidities. Emphasis on spirit rather than a body of knowledge makes overt that knowledge independent of a user is a non-sense.*

Recognizing that *knowledge is for use and consumption* is to stress that *the spirit of knowledge is needed throughout the ranks of the nursing profession.* This spirit of knowledge is not something that needs developing only in the academic elite of nursing. The suggestions we have given (see pp. 65–67, 71–72) about depersonalizing research and the move from competitive cooperation to a more genuine collaboration is a first step in moving toward a spirit of knowledge within that elite.

Still, that step is not enough. In what sense is that elite an elite? Only in the sense of having a primary obligation for cultivating the spirit of inquiry, not in having a corner on its skills or use.

Conversely, the practicing elite – the nurses in the real world of service – have a primary obligation for demanding relevance from their researching colleagues. Part of the blame – if one insists on talking in such old-fashioned guilt and sin terms – for any lack of practical significance from nursing research falls on the practitioners who scoff or withdraw rather than demand their rights as consumers. Could these practitioners not function to remove in part the hindrance to fruitful growth and use of inquiry in the ongoing practice of nursing? Away then with the priestesses of research as well as the ritual guardians of practice! On perhaps to a less secretive status-bound community of professionals!

What's Next?

In the spirit of the proposed openness, inquiry, too, should develop a new openness. Abandon the stance that searches out and wars over *the* definition of nursing, need, or empathy. Create the posture of tentative proposals with fruitfulness as measure and proposer as most willing critic. Clean-handed seeking for neat boundaries needs replacing by a more realistically oriented professional judgment about priorities.

Speaking in terms of priorities makes evident that the decisive judgments are subject to change and should be successively changed. Moreover, to speak of priorities rather than of the truth makes us ask, "Priorities for what?" Once we ask *that* question, we cannot easily evade the question of exactly how the activities carried on by persons claiming to be in the nursing profession are significant for nursing practice. This more earthbound orientation helps perhaps to direct even nursing *researchers* and *theoreticians* to a more finite time orientation.

To theorize and research in the hope and trust of an eventual payoff for nursing is ridiculous on two counts. First, given the pace of technological change, and hence of nursing practice and demands, long-term involvement in a search for delicately correct solutions to problems may well lead to solutions that appear only after the initiating problems have long since disappeared. No amount of self-righteousness about avoiding the mere problem-solving attitude to nursing research can cloak this feature of time pressure as highly pertinent, if any pretense at all is to be kept that theory or research has payoff for practice.

Such objective eternal verity–oriented research and theory is ridiculous on a second count. Such a stance overlooks the fundamental role of value or bias or goal orientation in any profession and hence in the inquiry for that profession. To pretend to be a nurse, to accept public health funding for nursing research, to regard nursing as a service, is ridiculous when conjoined to a claim that nursing priorities – the priorities of current nursing practice – do not have some *primary* relevance for both the priorities and methods of nursing inquiry.

This new posture or stance toward values we recommend without holy water or scriptures. The values need to be seen as pervasive and *now*-present guides to activity, not as eventual arrival points. The values need to be regarded as tentative and changeable rather than as almost religiously inviolable. And finally, they need to be regarded not as idols or starry dreams but as energy sources and steering devices.

Fixation, then, with the question of the proper structure of theory for nursing is not the only fixedness to be abandoned. We need to ask, "What's the use of theory?" in both senses of that question. Finesse with respect to structure of theory is a misplaced precision if the more general questions of integration and flexibility of theory and research with practice are left unconsidered. Talk of theory could be just so much irresponsible word play, draining energy from more suitable use and giving a false sense of security, hope, and justification – or merely a comforting sense of busyness.

POSTLUDE

Est-ce possible que les enfants sortiront jamais de l'église?
Peut être. Pourquoi pas? Les jeux y sont déjà faits. . . .

NOTES

Some further, more detailed points on which we would probably take some issue with Peplau's notions as given in the cited article are seen in the following letter, written to her on November 10, 1969. Hopefully, we try here for collaboration and not just competitive cooperation.

Dear Professor Peplau:

We have just had the good fortune to come across your article "Theory: The Professional Dimension," and we enjoyed reading it very much. We were, however, somewhat perplexed by the reference you made to one of our articles. You suggest we made a "glaring" omission. We are puzzled because we would not think of denying what you said we did deny – namely, "of using available concepts to name and thus to begin to explain observed phenomena and to derive theory-based nursing actions." Could you help us out? We heard you here in New Haven and were impressed by both your practicality and your general lucidity. Apparently our paper failed to communicate if even so astute a reader as you inferred we were denying the importance of using concepts whose referents were observable factors of the nurse-patient interaction, in the formation of nursing theory. Indeed, how did you understand the first level of theory that we isolated, namely, factor-isolating or naming theory? Why do you believe we called it first-level theory? We would genuinely like to know what gave rise to the misunderstanding: undoubtedly it is some flaw in the exposition, and since our aim is to communicate, you would do us a great service if you would bring us to an understanding of where our account went astray.

You quote Merton's view of science as involving "competitive cooperation." We find his notion too ascetic in the Nietzschean sense of asceticism, as Nietzsche explains that notion in his third essay in the *Genealogy of Morals*. Our next set of remarks is not offered in "competitive cooperation" but in genuine cooperation. That is, we find (1) errors and (2) unfortunate orientation in your essay. We bother to point them out to you, because we have a genuine interest in seeing progress made in the development of nursing theory and in the elevation of nursing to a professional status that allows it to function more efficiently and knowingly in the giving of nursing care. So, in this light, let us turn to the errors.

You are indulging in a logical blunder when you speak of deriving anything from concepts. You say "... choosing this concept [the concept of bleeding or hemorrhage], nursing interventions deriving from this concept are likely to follow." Logic traditionally distinguishes concepts from propositions. For example, a word 'prigs' expresses a concept, and a concept is not true or false. Similarly, a word 'philistines' expresses a concept. But the sentence "All prigs are philistines" expresses a proposition, i.e., a meaning which is either true or false. Now logic recognizes that from the concept in isolation nothing follows or can be derived, but from the proposition either in isolation or in conjunction with other propositions, an inference can be made. For example, from the proposition that all prigs are philistines can be derived the proposition that no prigs are nonphilistines, or, following the canons of traditional logic, the proposition that some philistines are prigs.

Strictly speaking, from the concept *bleeding* nothing follows. Clearly, what you intended was not what you said. The *concept* you probably had in mind was strictly speaking not a concept at all but a proposition that there is blood here. [Note that the distinction made here of concepts as opposed to propositions is made to clarify that from which derivation can occur; the usage suggested in this letter, then, is not precisely the usage we suggest in the present article, namely, that the proposition be regarded as a kind of concept. The purpose at present is to emphasize the sameness of ontological status as between concepts such as *bleeding* and propositions; in the letter, the emphasis is on showing what kind of "concept," namely, a proposition, is needed before derivation could be suitably talked about.] Now from this proposition in isolation very few interesting propositions can be derived. What is now required in your account is the articulation of how this proposition is supplemented with others to produce a deduction whose conclusion is a prescription that the nurse ought to do such and such. Another confusion exhibited in your essay is what philosophers call a mistake in ontology; that is, you confuse different realms of being. For example, you say, "Thus, the nurse who observes blood in some amount on the body and sheets of the bed of a patient, "flips up" a concepts such as *bleeding* or *hemorrhage*. . . ." Here the word 'concept' seems to refer to a mental act. On the other hand, you write a few paragraphs later: "On the other hand, a process represents many concepts which, taken together, provide explanations of a broader range of behavior. . . . A process is, in effect, an organization of concepts into large components – called phases, stages – each of which includes a series of separate concepts arranged in a serial order showing the emergence of particular behavior." Surely you do not mean a process is an organization of mental events (= concepts). In short, your exposition fails to distinguish between a concept as a mental event and that non-mental entity the concept refers to. Furthermore, if a concept is a mental event, how is it possible to speak of Nurse Mary and Nurse Jane having the same concept, namely, the concept *bleeding*? You might find modern logic helpful on these matters. Our *Symbolic Logic and Language* could be of some assistance to you; and we have detailed materials on the ontology of naming, concepts, definitions, etc., that you might find helpful. If you care to see them, we would be happy to send you a copy.

Now to the misorientation. If we understand you correctly, you conceive of theory simply as predictive theory. Predictive theory explains phenomena similar to the kind you now observe and you use this predictive theory to guide your choice in intervention in practice. But clearly, something more is needed. For suppose, for the sake of an example, it is a causal law that 15 minutes of bleeding at the observed rate will produce coma. What nursing intervention does that dictate? Is it always the case that as nurse you will want to prevent coma? What if the patient is terminal, aged, impoverished, etc.? The case is contrived because probably in most instances you as nurse act to sustain life. But the almost-alwaysness of a certain goal tends to obscure that the goal is there presumed in addition to the prediction in determining the nursing activity. Or more generally, what is needed to guide practice is 4th-level theory, which includes as one of its elements in the Survey List Ingredient predictive or third-level theory. But rather than labor the point more, we will stop now and await your reply. For we suspect that anything we might say with respect to situation-producing theory might continue to be in the same vein so esoteric in exposition as to continue to fail to communicate.

We do look forward to hearing from you.

With best wishes,

(signed) James Dickoff
Patricia James

On November 24, Professor Peplau replied that because of time limitations, she must postpone a definitive response to our letter.

REFERENCES

1. Wittgenstein, L. *Philosophical Investigations* (tr. by G. E. M. Anscombe). New York: Macmillan, 1953, p. 50e, par. 127.
2. Peplau, H. Theory: The Professional Dimension. In *Proceedings, First Nursing Theory Conference,* University of Kansas Medical Center, Department of Nursing Education, March 20–21, 1969, p. 34.
3. Dickoff, J., James, P., and Widenbach, E. Theory in a practice discipline. *Nursing Research* 17:415, 545, 1968.
4. Dickoff, J., and James, P. Theory of theories: A position paper. *Nursing Research* 17:197, 1968.
5. Dickoff, J., and James, P. Researching the role of research. *Nursing Research* 17:204, 1968.
6. Northrop, F. S. C. *The Logic of the Sciences and the Humanities.* New York: Macmillan, 1947, pp. 77–101. (For a related discussion)
7. Peplau, H., op. cit., p. 33.
8. Merton, R. K. Behavior patterns of scientists. *The American Scholar* 38:220, 1969.
9. Dickoff, J., and James, P. Societal Needs: A Basis for Curriculum Design. In *Proceedings of Duke University Symposium,* Aug. 25–29, 1969.
10. See page 1 of the *Proceedings* of the first of the three conferences, March 20–21, 1969.
11. See especially the *Proceedings* of the Third Nursing Theory Conference, January 29–30, 1970
12. The *Proceedings* for the three nursing theory conferences are dated respectively March 20–21, 1969; October 9–10, 1969; January 29–30, 1970.

13. See, for example, Dickoff, J., and James, P. Beliefs and values: Bases for curriculum design, *Nursing Research* 19:415–427, 1970.
14. For some considerations of the more unmentionable aspects of dynamics, see the paper cited in reference 13.
15. See, for example, *Proceedings of Second Nursing Theory Conference*, p. 68.
16. See Peplau, H., op. cit., p. 34.
17. See the paper cited in reference 13.
18. Russell, B. On Denoting. In H. Feigl and W. Sellars (Eds.), *Readings in Philosophical Analysis*. New York: Appleton-Century-Crofts, 1949.
19. See Dickoff, Jr., and James, P. Socrates – Still a Folk Hero for Education? in *Philosophy of Education: 1970*, Proceedings of the Twenty-sixth *Annual Meeting of the Philosophy of Education Society* for a discussion of the triad of speculators relevant for a practice discipline.

Behavioral Science Application in Nursing Research

II

THE three chapters comprising Part II are contributed by a nurse scientist and two social scientists collaborating with nurse investigators. The specific steps in the research process are presented in terms of the investigators' experiences in gathering and interpreting actual clinical data. Each chapter deals with the same basic problems encountered by nurse-investigators, but focuses on different aspects of the research process.

In Chapter 4, Doctors Leonard, Wooldridge, and Skipper relate behavioral science theory to practice theories encountered in nursing. Theories concerning stress are interwoven into a variety of clinical experiments originally conducted at Yale University School of Nursing. Patient-practitioner relationships and interactions are outlined. The designs of several experiments in the clinical setting of the hospital serve as guides for the conduct of similar investigations. The notion of the nurse as a dependent variable in patient stress is discussed.

In Chapter V, Doctors Leventhal and Israel cover conceptualization, observation, and analysis as related to the problems encountered by researchers in patient-response investigations. Measurement of variables in such studies is one of the most complex tasks nurse-investigators face, since both physiological and psychological responses are often intertwined. In the context of studies that illustrate the difficulties that are encountered, the authors discuss ways of tying these two kinds of clinical behavioral data together. A major portion of this chapter deals with different kinds of observation and the biases inherent in each. The handling of behavioral data is explained in terms of quantification, development of scales, and statistical treatment. Specific methods of assessing the realiability of behavioral measures is also presented.

Doctor Jeanne Quint Benoliel has derived from three investigations research experience helpful to other investigators. In the final chapter of Part II, she covers the research process in detail, with specific examples drawn from her studies of death and the dying patient, adjustment to mastectomy and the diagnosis of breast cancer, and of young diabetic patients learning the psychosocial meanings of their disease. These problems are extremely sensitive areas in our culture; therefore, additional problems and their solutions are outlined for the reader. Dr. Benoliel describes the role of participant observer in detail, particularly as related to the various steps in the research process, and discusses the conflict the clinical investigator faces between her role as nurse-practitioner and as objective researcher.

Ethical considerations and the confidentiality of clinical data are discussed by all of the authors as these relate to their own areas of research.

The Application of Behavioral Science to Patient Care as Illustrated by the Etiology and Control of Stress in Clinical Settings

Robert C. Leonard
Powhatan J. Wooldridge
James K. Skipper, Jr.

4

TO apply behavioral science theory to nursing means different things to different people. To us, it means a demonstration of how the insights available through these general theoretical perspectives can be used to improve the effectiveness of nurses in caring for patients. In this chapter, general behavioral science theory is used to interpret and integrate the results of a series of clinical experiments conducted by students and faculty at a school of nursing. The studies deal with a variety of clinical settings, investigative procedures, and symptomatology, but they all deal with a single major nursing problem: how to exercise effective control over the stress experienced by hospitalized patients. They all involve, as well, the use of sociopsychological treatment based on symbolic interaction. Proper understanding of this process involves the integration of social, psychological, and nursing perspectives through the application of social structural and symbolic-interactionist theory to the patient care system.

Until very recently, much of "nursing research" has been research about nurses. Such research is not designed to focus on a theoretical domain of inquiry uniquely oriented toward nursing. From a theoretical perspective, such research is no more *nursing* research than research into the motives and careers of biologists is *biological* research. In our view, the proper purpose of specifically *nursing* theory and research is to improve the effectiveness of nursing care of patients. We have called this theoretical domain or mode of inquiry "practice theory" [49, 50], and Maccia [45] has called it "praxiological" theory. Such theory and research deals with the effects of nursing means on nursing goals under conditions typical of nursing practice. But it does not call into question the worth of nursing goals, the rightness of restrictions on the means nurses are free to manipulate at their own discretion, or the moral appropriateness of the conditions under which nurses practice. These questions are matters of value that should be considered separately, as part of nursing philosophy, rather than as questions that can be decided by empirical research.

Given the existing practice of nursing, sociopsychological means have special relevance for the development of nursing theories of practice. When nurses administer medication, or when they use biological, chemical, or physical means in general, their authority is tightly circumscribed by the authority of physicians, and the scientific basis of their practice is derived largely from practice theories developed by the medical profession. In the use of psychosocial means to care for patients, however, nurses have a great deal of autonomy. Practice theories for the employment of such means of care have been largely neglected by the medical profession and by the behavioral sciences as well. Tests of hypotheses about the effects of social and psychological factors on the patient's physical responses to his illness would seem to be an obvious direction for medical sociology, as Kaplan and Bloom [20] have pointed out. But as their bibliography reveals, such research has yet to attract the attention of most medical sociologists. Furthermore, this aspect of nursing practice – the direct personal care of patients – is an area that nursing has traditionally acknowledged as its special province.

In the past, major obstacles to the development of scientific theories of practice in the sociopsychological area have been (1) failure to see the psychosocial aspects of care as appropriate subjects for scientific study and development ("patient care is an art, not a science"); (2) a failure to realize the full extent to which such factors influence the patient's physical response to medical treatment ("it's nice to keep the patients happy, but they're here for medical treatment, not to be pampered"); and (3) a tendency to see effective psychological manipulations as either incredibly difficult and risky ("I don't want any nurses trying to give psychological treatment to my patients"), impractical because of pressure on the staff ("our medical and nursing personnel are too busy to do a lot of hand-holding"), or extremely time-consuming ("solving a patient's psychological problems could take years!").

In recent years, these arguments have come to be recognized as half-truths and rationalizations with little or no validity. In study after study, nurses and other medical practitioners have demonstrated that major improvements in the patient's response to medical treatment can be produced by relatively simple changes in the psychosocial context of care. Far from being impractical and overly time-consuming, proper employment of such means can greatly improve the efficiency of cure, and in many cases even reduce the total amount of time spent in meeting patient demands.

The scientific evaluation of proposed means of meeting the patients' psychological needs has also begun to replace polemical assertions by advocates of one nursing approach or another. An important recent development is that well-designed experiments have begun to replace "demonstration studies" as the preferred means of testing the effectiveness of nursing procedures scientifically. Experimental research is the best way to evaluate effectiveness, and it is widely used in the medical setting to evaluate the efficacy of chemical and physical agents of control (drugs, for example). There has not, however, been a comparable emphasis on the use of experimental research to evaluate the effectiveness of social and psychological agents of control (communication between nurses and patient, or manipulation of the patients' definition of his situation, for example).

Many health practitioners have unrealistic stereotypes of

experimental research that discourage its use in this kind of application. On the one hand, many see experimental research in terms of the physics or biology laboratory, with extraneous variables controlled by holding them constant. Since such control would severely interfere with hospital routine, experiments are seen as impractical. This stereotype is not applicable to behavioral experimentation in which extraneous variables are permitted to vary, and randomization is used to insure that the effects of the extraneous variables are not systematically confounded (mixed in) with the effects of the procedure being evaluated. Such research is easily incorporated into the hospital routine and may even contribute to ongoing care at little or no cost to the clinical facility.

Other practitioners argue that ethical problems make experimentation with patients impossible. Such arguments ignore the fact that everything that nurses and other medical personnel do not do, as well as what they do, can have important effects on the patient's recovery. And in the absence of experimental verification, all psychosocial aspects of direct patient care are "experimental" in the sense that results are unpredictable and potentially harmful to the patient. Well-designed randomization experiments seem perfectly ethical when there is no rational basis for believing that inclusion in the study is more likely to harm than help the patient. Indeed, one might argue that it is failure to evaluate carefully the effectiveness of existing nursing procedures that is unfair to patients, and perhaps unethical as well.

We have argued that the behavioral sciences can make their greatest contribution to nursing through helping in development of practice theories [49]. We have argued that such theories should be tested experimentally, and that the results can make major contributions to the effectiveness of patient care. Finally, we have argued that the implementation of such a plan of theory building and research is technically feasible and not particularly difficult.

This chapter moves in that direction by expanding Orlando's [28] practice theory to include the sociological framework of patient-staff interaction. Orlando's theory was tested by faculty and graduate student research at the Yale School of Nursing.[1] We concentrate on an early (1961–1965) phase of experimental tests of the Orlando theory, partly because this is most pertinent to our general thesis and partly because it was this phase in which the authors were involved.

Social and Psychological Theories of Stress

Psychological symptoms of stress are important to nursing practitioners, and nurses have special skills in measuring and treating them. This provides an opportunity for nurses to undertake important sociosomatic research in the clinical setting. When properly conceptualized, such research can make important contributions to behavioral science theory and to nursing practice theory as well. At the same time, behavioral science theory can help to identify the etiology of stress and suggest ways to improve nursing care.

We will show (1) how structural inconsistencies can lead to kinds of staff-patient interaction that result in high levels of stress for clients and (2) how such stress can be controlled through restructuring nurse-patient interaction. We will then discuss the results of a number of previously published nursing studies in the light of this theoretical framework. The studies show some of the potential benefits to be derived from such sociopsychosomatic research, and they illustrate some of the ways the method of clinical experimentation can be used in various hospital settings.

As Martin [25] notes in his review of theories of stress, sociologists explain variations in stress behavior by variation in the integration of the social system. In macrotheory, status integration as a system characteristic has been used to explain suicide [15] and chronic illness rates [9]. In microtheory, status inconsistency or "crystallization" as an individual characteristic has been proposed as an explanation for behaviors ranging from self-isolation [22] through psychoneurotic stress symptoms [16, 17] to political rebellion [23, 32]. Psychological states such as anxiety, frustration, uncertainty, or stress have been hypothesized as intervening variables in both kinds of theory. In attempting to link the sociological and psychological levels of analysis, role conflict and role ambiguity have also been interpreted as aspects of social structural malintegration that have important effects on individual stress [19]. These theoretical interpretations have tended to converge with psychological theories of cognitive consistency [25].

The concept of "stress" has gained currency in several health-related sciences ranging from sociology through psychology to macrophysiology and microphysiology. It has been invoked by Dodge and Martin [9] to explain the rising chronic disease rates of modern societies and variations in these rates as a function of the integration of various status positions within a society. Cassell [5] notes that the failure of orthodox medical theory to explain variations in disease rates has led to "a reawakening of interest in the possible role of social and cultural stress factors as determinants of disease." Scott and Howard [33], in their review of stress theories, note different referents for the key term *stress.* They note that these "heuristic frameworks" that have emerged at various levels of analysis may be advanced to a comprehensive theory as new stress models emerge. Within nursing research, various terms have been used, including the near-cousin *distress.* In the interest of eventual linkage with other research work at other levels, however, we have decided to use the concept *stress*, recognizing that what we mean by stress will necessarily be somewhat different from the meaning in either macrosociological or microphysiological theories.

Cassell [5] comments that the hypothesis that stress affects health is not well handled by medical practitioners. It is not a useful guide to medical cure because the practitioner either does not know what to do about stress or else is not in a position to do anything anyway. For example, knowledge that the risk of lung cancer rises on moving to the city from the country does not lead to a practical prescription for either avoiding or curing lung cancer. Similarly, what can be done with the fact that upward social mobility appears to result in higher rates of many kinds of disease? Disease syndromes are probably the result of years of "sustained" social stress [9]. On the other hand, most of the stress research to date has focused on traumatic crisis events [33]. These results may fail to provide useful guidelines for dealing with the long-term health problems produced by chronic environmental stress, but they have major implications for dealing with temporary health problems caused by acute social environmental stress. And it is precisely such "situationally derived" needs [49] that are an important concern of nursing theory and practice.

Syndromes of patient condition involving accelerated heart rate, vascular contraction, facial perspiration, and the like are familiar signs for action to experienced nurses. Such symptoms suggest Selye's [34] concept of stress, but the situations in which they occur also suggest sociological notions of stress-producing inconsistencies in the social system. Furthermore, many nursing actions taken to relieve the symptoms appear strikingly consistent with sociopsychological theories of stress. If "patient condition" is recognized to be patient performance of the patient role, then the concept of equilibrium can be used to link the various levels of analysis.

A basic sociological insight is that the goal of the nurse in her interaction with the patient includes various kinds of social control. Not only does patient care aim to establish equilibrium within the patient, but it also aims to maintain equilibrium within the patient care social system. For example, both patient and nurse must follow hospital policy and must maintain good relations with the medical staff if system equilibrium is to be maintained. The concept of equilibrium subsumes the twin concepts of homeostasis and sociostasis. *Both* of these must be maintained if interaction between patient and nurse is to be truly effective. But, one may be maintained at the expense of the other, for example, patient stress may be tolerated, or even encouraged, in order to maintain system equilibrium. In such situations of conflict between sociostasis and homeostasis – between system and individual patient equilibrium – system change is necessary if undesired levels of patient stress are to be avoided. Of course, it is also possible to have conflicts due to malintegration within the system itself. For example, it may be necessary to remove some of the barriers to staff-patient communication in order to provide the patient with the information he needs to perform his role effectively.[2]

It is also possible that successful role performance in a crisis – and hospitalization itself is a crisis for a high proportion of patients – requires an optimal stress level: neither too much nor too little. Emotional support and accurate information about the situation from an authoritative source in the context of an expressive interaction may help regulate the individual's stress toward the optimum level.

Sociological Context of Patient Stress

In the modern hospital, potentially stressful situations are part of the daily routine. To a degree, stress is an unavoidable result of illness, and some stress may even promote therapy. But excessive and prolonged stress can be seriously detrimental to the patient's condition. A certain amount of stress may be all that gets most of us out of bed in the morning, but too much stress can cause us to stay there. When a person enters the patient role, he is likely to experience a considerable amount of stress due to malintegration in the network of role relations that makes up the social environment of the hospital. Literally, hospitals can produce illness symptoms.[3] This malintegration takes the form of role conflict, role ambiguity, and disjunctions between ends and means.

One source of role conflict in the patient lies in inconsistencies between the "patient" role and the "sick" role. Parsons [31] suggests that the "sick" role grants the privilege of relief from many obligations but adds the obligation of actively seeking to get well. However, when the sick person enters the hospital and becomes a "patient," he is systematically discouraged from actively participating in his own care and cure. More subtly, the sick role includes a right to receive solicitation and attention. To some extent, this conflicts with the low status accorded the patient role in the authoritarian hierarchy of the hospital. A crying child receives increased attention and care, but patient requests are called "complaints," and the staff tends to withdraw, both psychically and socially, from the complaining patient.

A related source of stress is role ambiguity. The patient tends to be depersonalized by the hospital staff. Patients are often thought of in terms of biopathological diagnostic categories, or administrative categories, or both, rather than as actors in a social system. Depersonalization combines with the conflict between the patient role and the sick role to produce uncertainty about the patient's rights and responsibilities [36]. This uncertainty promotes patient passivity and makes the staff hesitate to initiate interaction with patients except in task-related areas where rights and obligations are clearly defined by medical prescription and hospital policy. The resulting reduction in staff-patient communication may seem to lighten the load on the staff. However, lack of communication between staff and patients increases the probability of "deviant" patient behavior, such as uncooperativeness or the development of psychosomatic stress symptoms.

Another barrier to effective performance of the patient role lies in disjunctions between means and ends and between prescribed and proscribed means. Some of these are implicit in our consideration of the conflicts between the sick and patient roles. Passivity is thrust on the hospitalized patient partly by the staff's withholding information. Sometimes, information is withheld that the patient needs to determine his role obligations or to perform them successfully. Withholding information is not necessarily intentional on the part of the staff. It can result from the staff's ethnocentric assumption that the information important for performance of the patient role is the same kind of information needed for their own role. But whatever the reasons for withholding information, the consequence is a disjunction between the goals for which the patient is expected to strive and the means provided by the hospital system. The patient is expected to cooperate with the hospital staff in his care and cure, but he is denied access to necessary information about symptoms, treatment, and the hospital system.

Lenski's [22] concept of "status" crystallization appears relevant to an analysis of the patient's position in the hospital structure. This is particularly true of his reference to the consequences of poorly crystallized positions for the occupant's interaction with others:

> ... persons whose status is poorly crystallized constitute a social category peculiarly vulnerable to rebuffs, embarrassments, and disappointments ... more often denied rewards ... more likely to be subjected to disturbing experiences in the interaction process.

Lenski predicted social withdrawal as a consequence. In the hospital, if our description of the patient's position is correct, we would likewise predict patient retreat or withdrawal. A comparable examination of the staff's positions also leads to a prediction of their withdrawal from interaction with the patient. In fact, the predicted mutual withdrawal often does occur, and the patient becomes socially isolated [48]. Communication breaks down, with consequent pathologies, including a sort of patient paranoia that progresses in stages from the patient feeling that the staff does not care to a feeling of mistrust ("they make mistakes and are careless") and sometimes to an outright suspicion of a threatening conspiracy [41].

Contradictory, ambiguous role expectations and disjunctions between goals and means set structural limits to patient performance. These structural conditions are linked to performance by intervening stress states, which develop from conflicts between individual motivations and structural barriers [26]. "Normal" performance usually results from moderate stress. Either too much or too little stress tends to result in some form of deviant behavior. For example, in a study of surgical patients, Janis [18] concludes that individuals who manifest a very high level of preoperative anticipatory anxiety, or fear, or both, are particularly likely to experience fear of body damage after the operation. Patients who show a very low degree of anticipatory fear preoperatively tend to experience anger and resentment toward "danger-control authorities" postoperatively. The structural conditions of the situation may play a large part in determining the actual type of deviant behavior in a way analogous to Jackson's [16] different predictions of fight or flight responses depending on combinations of ascribed and achieved statuses. And there may be individual variation in the tendency toward such reactions. But all of them are nevertheless affected by the amount and content of staff-patient interaction.

Social Interaction to Control Patient Stress

Often the concept of patient role is limited to the patient-practitioner dyadic framework [29, 31]. This conception has been expanded by considering the organizational context of such patient-practitioner interaction [2, 36].

The relationship between a number of aspects of client-professional interaction can easily be misunderstood. Thus providing emotional support does not exclude professional detachment [35]. An instrumental approach to performing the expressive function in the system is both possible and desirable. This combination seems to come naturally to most (female) nurses, perhaps because instrumental manipulation via affective interaction is characteristic of the traditional female role in general. Emotional (affective) support for the patient can be provided while remaining affectively neutral, even on very intimate topics. This neutrality is facilitated, we suspect, by the specificity of the nurse-patient relationship. Many topics highly relevant to the purposes of nurse-patient interaction are usually regarded, outside of the hospital system, as intimate affairs only discussed in very close family or friendship relationships. Because of this similarity with close personal ties, such nurse-patient interactions might be interpreted as being diffuse. Yet, it is possible – and desirable in the patient-care context – to be both intimate and specific. Thus we can characterize nurse-patient interaction as specific, affectively neutral, and instrumental. Yet at the system level the nurse performs the expressive system maintenance function.

Being professional is, finally, distinct from being bureaucratic [44]. Professional detachment can lie in the neutrality of the professional's affective orientation, rather than in a bureaucratic-like remoteness or nonintimacy. In fact, bureaucratic authoritarianism can hinder or prevent performance of the expressive function by cutting off nurse-patient communication.

These considerations suggest a nurse-patient relationship that is expressive yet affectively neutral; person-oriented rather than task-oriented; nonauthoritarian; specific; and intimate. This may lie somewhere between a bureaucratic relationship and friendship. To perform the role effectively, the nurse explores the patient's feelings and the background of those feelings as possible causes of stress, no matter what topics it leads to – and these topics are very often ones that would be regarded as extremely intimate in everyday discourse and may even include some the doctor or hospital may prefer not be discussed, such as medical diagnosis, potential outcome of the treatment, or feelings toward the doctor and hospital.

The nurse-patient relationship is not a primary relationship. although neither is it secondary. The relationship is specific rather than diffuse. Discussions that might be appropriate for getting acquainted with a future friend may have little relevance to the professional role. In fact, irrelevant conversation is often a way of avoiding professional obligations rather than a way of discharging them. For example, in our experience, task-oriented, bureaucratic nurses sometimes raise tangential topics as a way of deflecting the patient's conversation away from difficult topics or presentation of emotional needs. This experience fits with Thorner's [42] observations of actual nurse role performance, even though it is different from the dominant professional ideology.

In considering the organizational context of the patient's interaction with hospital staff, we hypothesized a balance of forces in the patient's social environment – a sometimes very delicate balance, which, if upset, moves the patient away from effective performance of his role. Laboratory research shows that just one supporter can help an individual to maintain a realistic cognitive orientation under adverse circumstances [21]. This suggests that even a single supportive interaction with someone in the hospital might help the patient maintain the psychosocial balance necessary to his effective role performance. Our analysis of the role of the professional nurse implied that supportive interaction is one of the major responsibilities of her role. Our analysis of hospital structure showed that there are reasons why the likelihood that nurses or other hospital practitioners will actually give effective supportive care to patients is typically low. It follows that a significant reduction in the stress behavior of patients might be achieved by arranging for a "supportive" nurse to be part of the patient's hospital environment. Ideally, such a nurse would be functioning in a social context where she would be free of the typical structural constraints imposed by the hospital. In addition, she would have to have a reasonably high degree of communication skills and the motivation to apply these skills to provide supportive care.

To summarize our discussion to this point: Malintegration of the social system within which nurse and patient interact tends to result in (1) stress-provoking definitions of his situation by the patient and (2) somatic symptoms of this stress. Improved integration in the system, if the theory is correct, should result in reduced patient stress symptoms and thus in greater effectiveness and efficiency of the system.

Direct tests of this proposition were made by research nurses working from a special research role within the system. We will now review some of that research, which indicates that the immediate interactional context is more closely related to patient stress than is recognized in existing theory and practice, and that social sources of stress account for much of the variance in many somatic symptoms traditionally interpreted as the product of biophysical factors alone.

Some Experimental Studies

The basic design of the experiments was relatively simple. Nursing personnel are responsible for many of the "care" activities of the hospital, including admission procedures, presurgical care, care of women in labor, responding to patient complaints of pain, and a large number of other activities involving sets of repeated, similar patient-practitioner interactions. Thus the normal scheduling of the hospital can be used to provide samples of patients who are having similar kinds of experiences and who are being subjected to similar kinds of routines in similar physical environments. In addition, such samples are often reasonably homogeneous with respect to sex, type of medical treatment, age, and social background. While survey studies tend to stress representative sampling from essentially heterogeneous populations, experimental studies test hypotheses more efficiently if replications take place with a minimum of variation in antecedent variables. Under such conditions, sampling procedures tend to stress homogeneity, or even convenience, rather than unbiased representation of some larger population. When the major aim of the study is to test causal theory rather than to describe, such a "focused" sample is often the most appropriate choice. A basic strategy of experimental research is to run series of small sample experiments, each of which has high internal validity but doubtful external validity, and then to base claims to external validity on the cumulative results of all the experiments [49]. This is essentially the strategy that was adopted.

All the studies reported here were randomized experiments [14]. In each, the sample was randomly divided into "control" patients who went through the regular hospital routine; and "experimental" patients who interacted with a research nurse trained in techniques of supportive diagnosis and care. In some experiments, a research nurse was substituted for the staff nurse who would normally perform the task in question. In other experiments, the experimental patients received the full complement of routine service in addition to the special care provided by the research nurse. In both kinds of design, the experimental variable was conceived to be the supportive, nondirective, patient-centered role assumed by the experimental nurses.

The amount of stress experienced by the patients was measured in three ways: (1) through the reports of nurses and staff members, (2) through self-reports by the patients, and (3) through somatic indicators of stress. Reports by staff members and by the patients themselves are sometimes subject to bias even when single- or double-blind experiments are performed. In addition, it is not always possible to prevent the persons evaluating dependent variables from drawing some inferences about the probable purposes of the research or about the identity of experimental and control patients. We report here results only for those studies where it was possible to use somatic indicators of stress, such as increased blood pressure and pulse rate, temperature elevation, or postoperative vomiting. These kinds of behavior are only to a minor degree under the direct, conscious control of the actor. Thus, deliberate "overcooperation" on the part of the research subjects is minimized as a potential source of bias. Furthermore, somatic indicators are relatively easy to measure objectively. Insofar as this sort of information is routinely collected for hospitalized patients, these measures are largely nonreactive [46].

STRESS OF ADMISSION TO THE HOSPITAL

The entrance to any new social situation is very likely to be stressful since it entails disruption of normal anchorages for the individual's definition of his situation. The newcomer's needs for reassurance and information are implicitly recognized by many communities and organizations in their initiation and "welcoming" procedures. In contrast, the large urban teaching hospital is usually impersonal and oriented almost exclusively to biological needs in its admission of patients. Different phases of the patient's entrance are likely to be handled by a bewildering number of different aides, clerks, and nurses, each of whom has only a brief interaction with the new patient. Those interactions are usually task-centered, with a focus on medical condition and hospital routine, rather than on the patient's problem of adjusting to the new environment. The personnel carrying out the admission procedures tend to initiate interaction only when they need some data for their charts (e.g., financial standing, pulse, weight, temperature). When they speak, it is usually to ask for such information or to give orders about the specific task at hand. If a patient expresses distress, the staff are likely to respond with pleasantries about the weather or about some other tangential topic, or with a vague routine phrase of "reassurance." The typical role taken is the bureaucratic information-gatherer, chart-assembler, and order-deliverer. Somatic stress symptoms are either ignored or mistaken for disease symptoms that are only the concern of "the doctor."

The control patients in each of five experiments went through a regular admissions procedure. For comparison, a random half in each experiment were admitted by a research nurse who, in addition to performing the required tasks, found out how the patient was defining the experience and provided information and emotional support.[4] One experiment dealt with emergency room admissions to a general hospital, while a second dealt with admissions to a state mental hospital [1]. A third was concerned with scheduled admissions of clinic patients to a surgical ward. The other two experiments focused on scheduled admissions of private patients to a surgical ward [13]. In each study, blood pressure and pulse rates were measured for each patient both before and after the admission procedure. The difference between the patient's blood pressure before admission and his blood pressure after admission was interpreted as an indication of the amount of unrelieved stress concomitant with the admission process.

"Before" measures of blood pressure and pulse tended to be above normal levels in all of the experiments. They were most elevated for the emergency and mental hospital admissions (many came escorted by a policeman or in an ambulance with sirens screaming), less so for scheduled clinic (mainly lower-class) admissions, and least for private (middle-class) surgical admissions. As predicted, the experimental patients tended to show reductions in blood pressure and pulse rate. In contrast, the control groups tended to show either a *rise* or no change. Evaluations of stress based on posture, body movements, facial color, and facial expression corroborated the evaluations based on pulse and blood pressure.

The similarities in the results of these studies encourage confidence that admission to the hospital tended to produce stress and that the information and support provided by the experimental nurses tended to reduce stress in their patients. At the same time, there are some interesting differences in the results of the separate studies. The largest effect of the experimental interactions appeared to be with the emergency patients, the next largest with state mental hospital inmates, and the least with scheduled admissions of private surgical patients. This may have been due partly to variation in the initial levels of stress experienced by the different kinds of patients, since a higher initial level of stress provides the potential for a larger decrease. Internal analysis of the data indicates, however, that this was not the only factor operating.

In the emergency and mental patients, about one-half of the control patients displayed a *rise* in blood pressure during the admission procedure. This suggests that the relatively large between-treatment differences found in these experiments were due in part to stress induced by the hospital setting itself, which the experimental interaction counteracted. In contrast, only about one-fifth of the private surgical admissions experienced rises in blood pressure during the admission process. These private patients were entering a more orderly and well-staffed side of the hospital, where there may have been greater likelihood of stress reduction in the routine admission process. Thus the smallest experimental differences appeared where the social environment was already providing mechanisms for adjustment to the hospital. Perhaps these patients could use the assistance provided by the experimental nurse in adjusting to the situation, but lacking it, could actively seek and receive assistance from other sources. This interpretation is supported by the interview data. The private patients were asked whether they had been distressed on admission, whether that had been relieved, and if so, what had relieved them. Control group patients identified the admitting nurse as the source of relief less often than the experimental patients did, but that was balanced by relief from other sources in the hospital.[5]

Becoming a hospital patient entails separation from family and friends. If Parsons and Fox [30] are right, this contributes to family cohesion. But it can also increase stress for the individual and perhaps even for the family. This is especially the case when the patient is a child. Some hospitals recognize this by permitting parents to stay with young children who are hospitalized. This is seldom welcomed by the hospital staff. They now have a healthy, vertical, fully clothed adult to take into account – one who is competing or even conflicting with them in caring for the child. Having parents stay is a practical recognition of the fact that the parent is a highly important influence in the child's environment, whether or not the hospital personnel like it. But if the presence of the parent is to reassure the child rather than to alarm him, the parent must himself be calm and self-assured. Even while trying to avoid doing so, the parent can communicate his stress to the child involuntarily [37].

In three admission experiments, the sampling unit was expanded to include the parent – for all patients reported here, the mother [27, 38, 39]. Families with a child being admitted for tonsil-and-adenoid surgery went through an experimental admission process that included an expressive mode of response calculated to reduce the mother's stress and cognitive information to increase the mother's potential for effectively performing a supportive role in the hospital setting. Eight hours after surgery, the children in the experimental group averaged lower pulse rates than the children in the control group. In interviews at home with the mothers after the child's hospitalization, the experimental mothers reported fewer disturbances in the child's behavior, such as not eating and "being babyish." Throughout the course of hospitalization, the children in the experimental groups averaged significantly lower temperatures, pulse rates, and blood pressures. Similar differences appeared for in-hospital rates of postoperative emesis as rated by regular nursing staff and also for posthospital recovery as reported by mothers in mailback questionnaires [38, 39].

These results lend further strength to our theory that supportive, patient-centered interaction improves the patient's capacity to cope with potentially stressful situations, and that this improved capacity decreases somatic symptomatology. But admission to the hospital is far from the only stressful situation the patient is likely to encounter. If our general theory is correct, the stress-reducing effects of this type of interaction should be generalizable to other somatic indicators of distress and to other stressful situations.

THE STRESS OF SURGERY AND CHILDBIRTH

Surgery under general anesthesia is a serious procedure. Even when the surgical procedure itself is "routine," the anesthesia is always potentially hazardous. The progress of the patient is watched, often with tense anxiety by the staff, for signs of complications. Elaborate procedures are rigorously carried out to prevent such complications. The medical folklore recognizes the importance of patient "nervousness," and psychoanalysts have long emphasized that psychological states can have important effects on the results of surgery [7]. Yet many practitioners either remain unconvinced that postoperative complications can arise from preoperative stress, or rely on chemical means of stress prevention (such as tranquilizers), or else treat the symptoms rather than the stress itself (e.g., by prescribing antiemetics). Social and psychological means of stress reduction are usually given a low priority or ignored entirely. Practitioners sometimes even display a sort of moral indignation when a patient becomes highly distressed over what the staff define as being a "routine" operation [3].

Preoperative routines focus on the patient's physical preparation. These routines require the presence of many different specialists for varying lengths of time. But each specialist's orientation is focused on his own particular task rather than on the patient's definition of the situation. Even when the surgeon and anesthesiologist go out of their way to talk to the patient before the operation, they usually spend most of their time informing the patient about aspects of the surgery that are important to *themselves* in the performance of *their own role.* The patient is often left with no clear idea of how *he* is expected to behave.

Five experiments were designed to test the effects of expressive, patient-centered interaction on the amount of stress experienced by adult females scheduled for gynecological surgery. A random half of the patients on the operating schedule were assigned to interact with an experimental nurse who encouraged the patient to express and explore her reactions to the immediate situation and attempted to correct cognitive misunderstandings about the patient's role and about the possible consequences of the operation for the patient. Emesis in the recovery room was used as the major somatic indicator of stress.

In the first four experiments, the experimental nurse-patient interaction took place immediately before the operation. In two of these four experiments, additional interaction took place in the recovery room. For the total of 83 patients studied, the postoperative emesis rate was 54 percent for the control patients but only 16 percent for the experimental patients. Emesis was highly correlated with the research nurse's opinion of the patient's level of unrelieved preoperative distress and with the level of preoperative distress recalled by the patients in postoperative interviews [10]. The fifth experiment tested the effects of nurse-patient interaction at an earlier stage of the patient's hospital experience, just after surgery had been scheduled and before hospitalization. The results of this last experiment indicated little or no reduction in the postoperative emesis rate [11].

Our interpretation of these results is that (1) postoperative emesis is strongly affected by stress-producing factors in the immediate preoperative social environment; (2) the major effects of the kind of interaction introduced in these experiments are specific to immediate, situationally derived stress; and (3) the patient's ability to handle stress situations in the hospital is not likely to be permanently improved by a single supportive interaction, even though the effects on immediate stress can be great. Results from the admissions experiments with adult surgical patients previously cited, and from the experiments with child tonsillectomy cases, provide some support for this interpretation. In adult admissions experiments, where the supportive interaction with the patient occurred a considerable time prior to the operation, postoperative emesis rates were about the same for experimental patients and for control patients In the tonsillectomy experiments, where more or less continuous support was provided by the child's mother right up to the operation, the experimental group had a postoperative emesis rate of only 10 percent in comparison with a rate of 45 percent for the control group [24].

Psychosocial means tend to be emphasized much more in the care of mothers in labor than in the care of presurgical patients. Psychological, hypnotic, and other sorts of preparation for childbirth and support in labor often are advocated and actually practiced [4]. However, in spite of this relatively great emphasis on supportive care, much of the patient-staff interaction that takes place in the delivery room remains authoritarian and task-centered.

If our general theory is correct, then the physiological effectiveness of procedures that have somatic goals will be affected by the way the patient perceives his situation vis-à-vis the treatment procedure. This prediction was tested in two experiments with a predelivery enema routinely administered to women in labor. The stressfulness of the expectant mother's general situation, and the psychological and physiological discomfort usually involved in taking an enema, made this situation close to ideal for a test of the impact of the patient's definition of the situation on the degree of stress experienced. The experimental nurse attempted to obtain the patient's understanding and willing acceptance of the procedure by explicitly defining the patient's role as a cooperating participant, rather than an object of physical manipulation. In each case the experimental nurse waited until she had obtained the patient's consent before actually administering the enema. A nurse from the hospital staff administered the enema to the control patients. Analysis of the control interactions showed that the control nurses tended to depersonalize the interaction and to rely on authority to force the patient to comply with the treatment. As predicted, the effectiveness of the enema was significantly higher for the experimental patients, indicating a reduction in the stressfulness of the situation. The patient's verbal responses supported the interpretation that the experimental interaction had effectively reduced stress [43].

DISCUSSION

A basic sociopsychological proposition is that human action in a situation depends on the actor's definition of that situation. As sociologists, we conceptualize the somatic behavior of hospitalized patients as instances of individual human action, which can be affected by the patient's thoughts and feelings about his medical treatment and hospital care.[6] Another basic sociological proposition is that the actor's definition of his situation is changed through interaction with others. In the case of patient care, this means that psychological reactions and their physiological consequences are influenced by the patient's social environment.[7] This may seem like an obvious diagnosis to most sociologists, and in their review of the literature on stress theory, Dodge and Martin [9] were impressed by the minimization of physical sources of stress in favor of an emphasis on sociocultural factors. But, in fact, the sociocultural view of stress runs counter to much of current medical theory and practice. The impact of the patient's interaction with hospital personnel has received little recognition. In the variables regarded as important in setting up a medical service,[8] in the content of the practitioner's training [6], and in the medical researcher's selection of hypotheses to test, there has been a preference for a biological view of human nature, which has had the practical effect of neglecting social environmental sources of patient stress.

Sociologists often define sociology as the study of human interaction. But just as often we do not find it convenient in our research to observe interaction, or, for that matter, the actual behavior that is supposedly affected by interaction. Usually, self-reports seem more accessible for study. Sociologists have accumulated data suggesting that status inconsistency, or low status crystallization, is likely to go with liberal political attitudes, voting for the Democratic party, or – depending on the kind of inconsistency we are talking about – a higher frequency of self-reported psychosomatic symptoms. As far as we can determine, this line of research is not explicitly linked to the "social structure and anomie" theories of deviant behavior stemming from Durkheim [12], but it has been linked to the "status integration" and suicide research that also derives from Durkheim and with psychological theories of cognitive dissonance [25]. Previous sociological research has relied primarily on static macrolevel correlations, using census-type statistics for infrequent events such as suicide; or on survey analyses of self-reported physiological and psychological stress symptoms correlated with various indices of individual status consistency. The intervening social process activating the stress has not figured explicitly in the research, and the research has not been experimental.

The data we have discussed differ from the sort of research results commonly brought to bear on social stress theory in at least three important ways: (1) they are the result of controlled experimentation; (2) they deal primarily with somatic indicators of stress; and (3) they involve interacting dyads as the basic unit of analysis. This kind of research provides a level of internal validity for causal interpretations not readily obtainable through macrolevel correlations or when stress is measured by responses to a questionnaire.

Our general interpretations of the results of the research can be summarized as follows: (1) The amount of stress experienced by an actor in a situation depends to a large extent on the actor's definition of the situation. (2) The actor's definition of the situation often depends on the context and content of his interaction with significant others immediately prior to and during the occurrence of potentially threatening stimuli. (3) Many somatic behaviors not usually considered to be under the actor's conscious control are nonetheless strongly influenced by the actor's definition of his situation. More specifically, the depersonalization of the patient that prevails in many hospital situations tends to result in (1) largely nontherapeutic interactions between patient and staff; (2) stress-provoking definitions of his situation by the patient; and (3) a great amount of somatic symptomatology. Under these circumstances, interaction with a health practitioner trained in techniques of effective communication can result in large reductions in the stress experienced by the patient and in a large decrease in somatic complications. The size and consistency of the experimental effects obtained in the research indicates that the immediate interactional context of stimuli is more closely related to the production of stress than is usually recognized, and that sociopsychological stress accounts for much of the variance in a variety of somatic behaviors usually interpreted as the product of biophysical factors.

ACKNOWLEDGMENTS

This paper draws heavily on our experience with the Yale School of Nursing research program, which owes its inception and continuation to many more persons than could possibly be mentioned here, although the work of many of them is cited at appropriate points in the text. In addition, we should acknowledge the contributions of our nursing colleagues at the universities of Arizona, and Western Ontario. The writing benefited from comments on an earlier draft by R. F. Curtis. Financial support has included grants and fellowships from the Commonwealth Fund, American Nurses Foundation, and United States Public Health Service including Grants GN-88833, NU-00060, and Yale Medical School Grant PHS1-401-FR-05358-01.

NOTES

1. The dominant orientation of the school was a version of Sullivanian psychoanalytic theory, with an intense commitment to direct patient care in a context of strong research expectations from the university administration. Within a period of five years, a loosely formulated theory of nursing had been developed and was being taught. (See Orlando [28] and Wiedenbach [47]. See also F. S. Wald and R. C. Leonard, Toward nursing practice theory, *Nursing Research,* 13:309–313, 1964; F. S. Wald, Emerging nursing practice, *American Journal of Public Health* 56:1252–1260, 1966.)

2. Exactly the same analysis could be applied to performance of the nurse's role. System equilibrium maintained at the expense of undesirable levels of nurse stress also reduces system effectiveness and efficiency.

3. It may seem unnecessarily iconoclastic or cynical to suggest that hospitals make people sick. But before the days of asepsis, this was a biological reality that is now acknowledged, and there is reason to suspect that this is still true for social environmental sources of symptoms (for example, see Deane [8]).

4. Memory reconstructions of nurse-patient interactions from one experiment showed that the control nurses dominated the interactions, talking more than the patients and using commands five times more often than the experimental nurse [43]. The experimental approach was less directive, giving the patient a chance to express reactions to the procedure. In only 2 of the 25 interactions did the control nurses use open-ended questions more often than closed ones. In contrast, in 18 out of 25 cases, the experimental nurse asked more open-ended questions. The median was 8 percent open-ended questions

by the control nurses and 54 percent by the experimental nurse. The higher proportion of open-ended questions in the experimental interactions suggests an approach aimed toward information-getting and increased patient participation.

Of course, many of the most important differences are communicated nonverbally and thus are not likely to show up in verbal records. At this point our only conclusion is that much additional research is needed before more precise specification of the independent variation will be possible. Research in a laboratory, in clinical settings where there is less noise, or where interaction is verbal, such as home visits by public health nurses, may be required. Neither memory reconstructions, tape recordings, nor stenographer's notes appear to provide complete or unbiased records. However, considerable fuzziness in the independent variable can be tolerated in the early stages of research of this kind. Our experiments should be replicable with even less specification of the independent variation than we provide in this report. At the very least, the experiments show that social interaction does have important effects on the patient. The implications of this for patient-care research, if not directly for current practice, are far-reaching.

5. In addition, there are two nontheory explanations (1) measurement of the dependent variable was "blind" in only the fourth experiment. Thus, correlated measurement bias remains a possible explanation for the observed differences in the first three experiments. Although blood pressure and pulse rate seem very easily standardized and easily objectified, in contrast to most sociological measurements, there remains room for observer bias. Although in further replications this possibility should be prevented by blind procedures, it is not likely that the differences in the magnitude of the apparent effect of the nursing treatment could be accounted for by differences in measurement bias from experimenter to experimenter. (2) Of course, as with even the most rigorous scientific probability inference, there remains a remote chance that the outcomes are simply random fluctuations.

6. It is at this point that the sociologist is likely to part company with many of his medical colleagues. Their implicit biological determinism limits their willingness to entertain the possibility that the individual can exercise control over such reflexes. At the same time, medical sociologists have not rushed to challenge this biological determinism. It is precisely with these kinds of hypotheses that the most crucial tests can be made of the two competing orientations. (Compare Martin's [25] suggestion of the potential in physiological measures.)

7. Having already parted company with most medical researchers at this point, the sociologist is likely to do so with many psychologists and psychiatrists who will judge these psychological factors to be matters of personality requiring long-term therapy and not something that can be readily modified in the immediate preoperative period.

8. In a forward-looking architectural book on the design of surgical suites, there are frequent but extremely brief and vague references to the "psychological effects" of "the environment" on the patient. The vagueness of these

references is in sharp contrast to the very explicit references to ancillary spaces for the comfort and relaxation of the staff, such as surgeon's change room, lounges, coffee room, and so forth [40].

REFERENCES

1. Anderson, B. J., Mertz, H., and Leonard, R. C. Two experimental tests of a patient-centered admission process. *Nursing Research* 14:151–157, 1965.
2. Bloom, S. W. *The Doctor and His Patient: A Sociological Interpretation.* New York: Russell Sage Foundation, 1963.
3. Brown, E. L. Meeting patient's psychosocial needs in the general hospital. *The Annals of The American Academy of Political and Social Science* 346:123–124, 1963.
4. Buxton, L. *Psychophysical Methods for Relief of Childbirth Pain.* Philadelphia: Saunders, 1962.
5. Cassell, J. Physical Illness in Response to Stress. In S. Levine and N. A. Scotch (Eds.), *Social Stress.* Chicago: Aldine, 1970.
6. Daniels, M. J. Affect and its control in the medical intern. *American Journal of Sociology* 66:261, 1960.
7. Davidson, H. Emotional precipitation of death. *Journal of the Medical Society of New Jersey* 46:350, 1949.
8. Deane, W. M. The reactions of a nonpatient to a stay on a mental ward. *Psychiatry* 24:61–68, 1961.
9. Dodge, D. L., and Martin, W. T. *Social Stress and Chronic Illness: Mortality Patterns in Industrial Society.* South Bend, Ind.: University of Notre Dame Press, 1970.
10. Dumas, R. G., and Leonard, R. C. The effect of nursing on incidence of postoperative vomiting. *Nursing Research* 12:12–15, 1963.
11. Dumas, R. G. Nursing preparation of patients for hospitalization and surgery. Mimeographed. New Haven, Conn.: Yale University School of Nursing. Interim report to United States Public Health Service, grant NU00060-0409 (1966).
12. Durkheim, E. *Suicide.* Glencoe, Ill.: Free Press, 1951.
13. Elms, R. R., and Leonard, R. C. Effects of nursing approaches during admission. *Nursing Research* 15:39–48, 1966.
14. Fisher, R. A. *The Design of Experiments.* Edinburgh: Oliver and Boyd, 1935.
15. Gibbs, J. P., and Martin, W. T. *Status Integration and Suicide.* Eugene: University of Oregon Press, 1964.
16. Jackson, E. F. Status consistency and symptoms of stress. *American Sociological Review* 30:556–564, 1965.
17. Jackson, E. F., and Burke, P. J. Status and symptoms of stress: additive and interaction effects. *American Sociological Review* 30:556–564, 1965.

18. Janis, I. *Psychological Stress.* New York: Wiley, 1958, Chap. 26.
19. Kahn, R. L., Wolfe, D. M., Quinn, R. P., Diedrick, J., Snoek, X., and Rosenthal, R. A. *Organizational Stress: Studies in Role Conflict and Ambiguity.* New York: Wiley, 1964.
20. Kaplan, H. B., and Bloom, S. W. The use of sociological and social-psychological concepts in physiological research: a review of selected experimental studies. *Journal of Nervous and Mental Disease* 130:128–134, 1960.
21. Krech, D., Crutchfield, R., and Ballachey, E. *Individual in Society.* New York: McGraw-Hill, 1964, pp. 507–515.
22. Lenski, G. E. Social participation and status crystallization. *American Sociological Review* 21:458–464, 1956.
23. Lenski, G. E. *Power and Privilege.* New York: McGraw-Hill, 1966, pp. 86–88.
24. Mahaffy, P. R. The effects of hospitalization on children admitted for tonsillectomy and adenoidectomy. *Nursing Research* 14:12–19, 1965.
25. Martin, W. T. Socially induced stress: some converging theories. *Pacific Sociological Review* 8:63–69, 1965.
26. Merton, R. K. Social Structure and Anomie. In *Social Theory and Social Structure.* Glencoe, Ill.: Free Press, 1956, pp. 131–194.
27. Moran, P. A. Parents in pediatrics. *Nursing Forum* 2:25–37, 1963.
28. Orlando, I. J. *The Dynamic Nurse-Patient Relationship.* New York: G. P. Putnam's, 1961.
29. Parsons, T. *The Social System.* Glencoe, Ill.: Free Press, 1951, Chap. 10.
30. Parsons, T., and Fox, R. Illness, therapy and the modern urban family. *The Journal of Social Issues* 8:2–44, 1952.
31. Parsons, T. Definitions of Health and Illness in the Light of American Values and Social Structure. In E. G. Jaco (Ed.), *Patients, Physicians and Illness.* Glencoe, Ill.: Free Press, 1958, pp. 165–187.
32. Rush, G. B. Status consistency and right-wing extremism. *American Sociological Review* 32:86–93, 1967.
33. Scott, R., and Howard H. Models of Stress. In S. Levin and N. A. Scotch (Eds.), *Social Stress.* Chicago: Aldine, 1970.
34. Selye, H. *The Stress of Life.* New York: McGraw-Hill, 1956.
35. Simpson, R. L., and Simpson, I. H. Women and Bureaucracy in the Semi-Professions. In A. Etzioni (Ed.), *The Semi-Professions.* New York: Free Press, 1969.
36. Skipper, J. K., and Leonard, R. C. *Social Interaction and Patient Care.* Philadelphia: Lippincott, 1965.
37. Skipper, J. K., Jr. Mothers' distress over their children's hospitalization for tonsillectomy. *Journal of Marriage and the Family* 28:145–151, May, 1966.
38. Skipper, J. K., Leonard, R. C., and Rhymes, J. Child hospitalization and social interaction: an experimental study of mothers' feelings of stress, adaptations and satisfaction. *Medical Care* 6:496–506, 1968.
39. Skipper, J. K., and Leonard, R. C. Children, stress and hospitalization: a field experiment. *Journal of Health and Social Behavior* 9:275, 1968.

40. Smith, W. *Planning the Surgical Suite.* New York: F. W. Dodge Corporation, 1960.
41. Tagliacozzo, D. L. The Nurse from the Patient's Point of View. In J. K. Skipper and R. C. Leonard (Eds.), *Social Interaction and Patient Care.* Philadelphia: Lippincott, 1965, pp. 211–222.
42. Thorner, I. Nursing: The functional significance of an institutional pattern. *American Sociological Review* 20:531, 1955.
43. Tryon, P. A., and Leonard, R. C. A clinical test of patient-centered nursing. *Journal of Health and Human Behavior* 7:183–192, 1966.
44. Vollmer, H. M., and Mills, D. L. *Professionalization.* New York: Wiley, 1966.
45. Walker, L. O. Toward a clearer understanding of the concept of nursing theory. *Nursing Research* 20:428–435, 1971.
46. Webb, E., Campbell, D., Schwartz, R., and Sechrest, L. *Unobtrusive Measures: Nonreactive Research in the Social Sciences.* Chicago: Rand McNally, 1966.
47. Wiedenbach, E. *Clinical Nursing: A Helping Art.* New York: Springer, 1964.
48. Will, G. T. A sociopsychiatric nursing approach to intervention in a problem of mutual withdrawal on a mental hospital ward. *Psychiatry* 15:193, 1952.
49. Wooldridge, P. J., Skipper, J. K., Jr., and Leonard, R. C. *Behavioral Science, Social Practice, and the Nursing Profession.* Cleveland: The Press of Case Western Reserve University, 1968.
50. Wooldridge, P. J. Metatheories of nursing. *Nursing Research* 20:494–495, 1971.

The Behavioral Measure: Conceptualizing, Researching, and Analyzing Psychological Factors in Nursing Research

Howard Leventhal
Sherry Israel

5

EVALUATION is a central issue for any practice discipline. Articulate and self-conscious members of the group will question whether their actions have the positive effects ascribed to them. This question is the first step toward controlled experiments, which in nursing would ask for a comparison between patients given special, experimental nursing (the experimental group) and patients who receive a different or standard type of nursing (the control group).

Having grasped the need for a controlled comparison, the questioner will then ask "On what criteria can I compare my groups? What effects should I expect? How can I record them? Can they be treated quantitatively, and can I draw reasonable conclusions about my treatments?" In this chapter we shall discuss a variety of problems involved in answering these questions.

The problems fall into three major classes:

1. Conceptualization: what one wishes to know about the patients' behavior, and how to define it in observable and measurable terms.
2. Observation: how to record the behaviors; and the various sources of error or confusion in different observation procedures.
3. Analysis: the examination of data and the preparation of scores and the implications of these steps for statistical description and inference.

The main focus of this chapter, therefore, is on the researcher's problems with dependent variables; the choosing, recording, coding, summarizing, and scoring of behavior, whether verbal, expressive, or autonomic. The main lesson, however, is this: solutions to each of the separate problems are interdependent, and the interdependence derives from the researcher's theory and the particular question she is asking about the underlying processes affecting the patient's response to treatment.

The typical treatise in this area is organized around a variety of issues relating to scaling and measurement; e.g., measurement scales (categorical, ordinal, interval, and ratio) and the reliability and validity of measures. This material is important, and we shall cover much of it here, but there will be important differences.

First, rather than organizing our presentation in terms of the logic of measurement or the logic of statistics, we are ordering it in terms of the logic of research and following the sequence in which such questions usually arise in experimental and observational studies, namely, the sequence of conceptualization, observation, and analysis. Second, we will focus on problems of research procedure and cover topics usually omitted in texts on statistics or experimental design. Third, we have selected problems in each of the three areas of conceptualization, observation, and analysis that seem especially relevant to the measurement of patient response to nursing treatments.

Some of the emphasis reflects our experience as investigators, teachers, and reviewers of the experimental work of students and colleagues; we want to attack the more frequent problems. Thus some of our discussion could be useful to the experienced investigator. But we address ourselves mainly to the beginning researcher, the person who has some familiarity with elementary statistical tools but could benefit by knowing in advance the pitfalls in the application of research design, the development of data collection devices, and the summary and analysis of data.

Success in dealing with conceptualization, selection of measures, procedures for observation, and analysis is an important determinant of the success of any research project. Elegance of experimental design will not make up for failures to define and measure the relevant behavioral indicators properly. It is apparent even in the leading contemporary journals of personality and social psychology that many students of human behavior are far more expert in inventing clever and occasionally well-controlled situations to manipulate action than in devising measures of relevant behavioral consequences. Several investigators [67, 75] have commented on this point.

The patient-care setting provides a unique opportunity to focus on extremely important classes of human behavior. The nurse-researcher can therefore contribute both to the advancement of nursing and to our basic understanding of human action. For the nurse-researcher to make the most of this opportunity, it is important to recognize that general and remote criteria, such as recovery from illness, are insufficient to evaluate and test nursing processes. Such a criterion is simply too remote in time to record the effects of the many specific aspects of treatment; and, like other such criteria, its value is dependent on a host of intervening steps. A major goal for research, therefore, will be the establishment of criteria more proximate to the treatment; the more proximate a criterion to a nursing activity, the more likely is any relationship between them to prove "lawful" and repeatable [15].

By recognizing the need for more accurate criteria, we assume the task of developing a more general model of the treatment process. Without such a model the research will seem piecemeal and insignificant, as it will be impossible to interrelate studies of the effects of specific nursing practices on specific criteria. In the context of a model of the movement from illness through treatment to recovery, the separate studies become meaningful contributions to the understanding of the specific processes occurring at particular points in time and in relationship to one another. The result is a map detailing the complex route to recovery.

THE PROCESS OF CONCEPTUALIZATION

Theory and Selection of Measures

The investigator's theoretical concepts are her single most important guide for the choice of behavioral measures. The goals of nursing include statements of relatively abstract psychological concepts; e.g., reducing the patient's *emotional distress,* or providing the patient with a *sense of control* so that he may make *rational choices* about his future. Discussions of the psychological concepts of distress, choice, autonomy, and so on, fill whole chapters, even books, and subsume a number of complex theoretical models that describe processes taking place during distress, choice, or autonomy. These concepts and their models coordinate with specific environmental and behavioral events, the specifics that ground or operationalize the model in a network of observables.

The table provides an overview of the steps involved in moving from a general problem to the test of a specific experimental hypothesis. One begins with the overall problem, such as decreasing anxiety at admission [2] or reducing patient pain, and attempts to develop a preliminary model of the theoretical process involved in anxiety, distress, or pain reduction. This model will then lead to operational definitions; that is, it will point to links between concepts and antecedent environmental conditions and between concepts and behavioral measures. The utility of the concepts in the model is related to their ability to point to their specific environmental antecedents and behavioral consequences.

While there must be public agreement as to which acts and environmental antecedents are the referents for the process, it is important to recognize that the referents are not equivalent to the process. Thus an investigator may define anxiety in terms of

Table. From Problem, to Concept, to Operations, to Analysis

I. Conceptual Formulation
  A. Problem definition: Effects of stress on adaptation and recovery
  B. Process model

Time 1		*Time 2*		*Time 3*		*Time 4*
Internal and external cues	→	Classified as signs of danger	→	Evaluation of cause and severity ↓	→	Coping Resources Plans ↑
				Emotion, fear, anger, hopelessness		

II. Operation Definitions
  A. Antecedent conditions: nonmanipulated
    1. Environmental stressors
      Type of surgery, medication, staff treatment, complications, proximity to surgery
    2. Subject factors
      Social class: education, finances, cultural factors, prior hospitalization, knowledge of illness
  B. Antecedent conditions: manipulated
    1. Type of nursing care
      a. Constant components: aimed at physical needs
      b. Variable components: aimed at affect reduction
  C. Dependent variables
    1. Attitudes and affect
      a. Verbal measures
        Mood and emotion
        Attitude toward staff: criticalness versus acceptance
      b. Behavioral measures
        Expressive signs: restlessness, eating
        Physiological signs: heart rate, sweating, etc.
    2. Coping
      a. Verbal measures
        Plans for the future
        Types of information sought
      b. Behavioral measures
        Days in hospital, time in bed versus ambulating, resuming pre-illness tasks (dressing self, etc.), requests for medication

III. Analysis and Verification: Relationships of Dependent Measures to Antecedent Factors
  A. Summary of data (descriptive statistics) and analysis (statistical testing) with careful attention to confounding factors and to artifacts of interval size, etc.
  B. Relationships to manipulated factors: test hypotheses and confirm conceptual validity of measures
  C. Relationships to nonmanipulated factors: can support conceptual validity of measures and can help rule out influences of irrelevant factors that may confound data

respiration rate or in terms of verbal reports of fear [22] and assume that these public representations actually reflect changes in anxiety. But since these are only measures and not actually the process, the investigator must recognize that a wide variety of behaviors might be equally good or even better representations of the process.

For example, besides respiration, our measures of anxiety could include heart rate, palmar sweat, and complaining. The selection of measures is further complicated by the fact that the functioning of even a single organ can be measured in many ways; e.g., for the heart, we can measure beats per minute, blood pressure(s), or pulse volume.

Variations in recorded behavior may stem from many sources other than just the process under study. For instance, change in heart rate may indicate a patient's distress, but it may also reflect physical effort or excitement at good news. The same applies to facial expressions such as frontalis muscle contractions [59]. The operational measure is sensitive to a broad range of processes in addition to those included in the process under study.

The researcher must have this clearly in mind before she designs and executes the study. Once she has collected the data, it is too late to realize that the record of respiration informs us about the breathing rate, but gives an inadequate and possibly misleading picture of the patient's emotional status. The record of any single behavior does not represent the richness of the behavior pattern so obvious to the casual observer. This would not matter if the measure used related perfectly to the psychological concept being investigated. Since it does not, the investigator must ask whether her behavioral record will have the information necessary and sufficient to reflect the process under study.

There is one important feature to the measurement of a psychological or behavioral process that is often less apparent (though it is equally present) in other scientific investigation. Because any behavioral measure can reflect a number of underlying processes, the actual meaning of the observation, the determination of what is causing variation in the measure, is tied to the context of observation and to the design of the experiment. Thus, heart rate is heart rate and reported pain reported pain. Whether variation in these responses reflects mediating processes of emotional distress, sensory pain, or brain damage can only be determined in the context of observation. A patient in the dentist's chair may report pain, show heart rate acceleration, and wince, either because the Novocain needle hits the facial nerve (sensory pain), or because he is emotionally upset by the dentist's remarking that he will lose his two front teeth (emotional distress). Heart rate may fluctuate during a decision to undergo surgery (anticipatory fear) or during the effort to walk after surgery (pain plus distress).

Experimental designs represent efforts to increase understanding of the processes that mediate behavioral changes. Experiments have two critical advantages over ordinary observations: (1) specification of the conditions for observation, and (2) inclusion of several conditions for observation (usually selected to differ from one another in relatively simple and well-defined ways). Thus an experiment may compare two treatments differing in only one way (the visible presence or absence of the nurse), or may compare two different variables of treatment simultaneously (visible presence and verbal communication) in a four group design. The experiment is the visible embodiment of the antecedent conditions and behavioral measures that define the theoretical process and thus allows us to attribute changes in observed behavior to specific environmental events.

If the problem under study has a long history, the theories available to the investigator will not only suggest concepts and measures but also potential relationships between concepts. For example, Tomkins [86] proposed that high levels of continuous stimulation produce distress, but that at very high levels of stimulation the distress may be replaced by anger. Therefore one might expect fluctuations of distress and anger, depending on the onset, duration, and intensity of stimulation. If epinephrine output were our only measure of disturbance, we might find increases in this adrenal hormone closely related to other measures of distress. But if Tomkins is correct, at very high levels of stimulation we should find increases in norepinephrine with little increase or even a decrease in epinephrine production. This shift in pattern among the biological measures could reflect a change from distress to anger, as anger is associated with a relatively high norepinephrine output [6, 78]. To avoid mistaking all shifts in epinephrine level as reductions in distress, the investigator must either anticipate the occurrence of anger and use some other measure to detect it, or regularly include other measures on the general intuition that she might uncover such effects.

Theory therefore guides the investigator, pointing to a variety of processes that might confound her observations and suggesting measures to detect these processes in order to separate their influence from that of the process directly under study. She thus obtains a coherent pattern and can distinguish the relevant from the confounding process. The pattern, or consistency of relationship among measures, establishes the validity of the investigator's theoretical constructs [14, 17].

Measuring at Multiple Levels

Organisms respond as complex units. When a person reacts with fear, anger, shame, distress, or joy, he has different subjective experiences, looks different, and may react differently internally. This means that the intervening emotional process can be operationally defined at many levels. Let us take discomfort as an example. When a person is uncomfortable, he usually knows it and can verbalize the feeling if asked to do so [21, 40]. Thus the cognitive or thought responses of the individual provide data for defining discomfort. But discomfort alters expressive and motor behavior as well as thought; in pain, the forehead and eyes are particularly likely to change appearance [31, 59], and the face will show an unpleasant expression [24, 94]. These, and many other aspects of motor behavior, such as thrashing of the arms, tension in specific muscle groups, and twisting of the trunk, could serve as distress measures. In addition, there are various internal measures of distress such as heart rate and blood pressure; rapidity, depth, and smoothness of breathing; and the electrical activity of the skin.

Since she can record behaviors at each of these levels, how can the investigator decide which response is the best measure? Many questions arise at this point, but we shall consider only three: (1) Is the physiological level of response a better measure of reactions than motor or verbal responses? (2) Should several measures be taken across and within levels? (3) What should be done if different levels disagree with one another?

WHICH LEVEL IS MOST BASIC?

In our culture, a strong bias exists toward psychophysical dualism, the view that mind and body are separate yet interacting entities. Associated with this view is a bias toward physical explanation; many consider physical causes more basic than psychological causes. This view assumes a hierarchy of explanations: if we know the physiological processes that accompany a behavior, we may think we have all the information needed to understand the behavior's "causes" and consequences. The bias toward physiological explanation also tends to assume that physiological responses are predictable and regular, while psychological behaviors (e.g., choices, likes) are unreliable, if not entirely random.

While it is true that psychologists, biologists, and chemists look at different aspects of behavior and conceptualize what they see in different ways, none of these conceptualizations is more "real" than any other, nor is any intrinsically more trustworthy or unreliable. All scientists abstract from the phenomenon under observation and construe it in ways appropriate to their different purposes. These constructions are supplementary rather than interchangeable, and they do not form a hierarchy of "goodness," where more basic explanations can substitute for less basic ones. For example, when a patient rings for the nurse, we could describe this activity in terms of the patient's motivations for ringing (that is, the aim or the effect he hopes to produce in the environment), the act of ringing (the movements of the body and the arms [89]), or the physiological events at the cellular or molecular level during this activity. Each of these descriptions can be objective, i.e., public and reliable, and each tells us something different about the action. However, if an investigator believes that the process she is studying affects behavior at different levels (e.g., distress is felt, reflected in muscular tension and autonomic response), she has good reason to attempt measurement at each level, since *convergence between measures* (correlations between them for several patients at a common point in time, or correlations within patients over several points in time) provides strong evidence for the concept under study [14]. In addition, the presence of specific physiological effects with a particular psychological state may have important implications for medical treatment.

But as our earlier discussion suggested, the investigator cannot typically use physiological measures to describe the consequences of various nursing practices, as these measures relate to multiple processes. Shapiro and Crider [81] have stated this point very well:

> In the most concrete sense, physiological variables are measures of nothing but themselves, and cannot be taken as ready-made indicators of sociopsychological constructs. A response measure, whether of overt or covert functioning, has meaning only in the context of observation.

HOW MANY MEASURES?

Measures at more than a single response level have been recommended, but how many measures should we use? If we use two and find they are highly correlated, we have probably identified measures of a common concept.[1] What if the two do not relate? Possibly either or neither measure is an indicator of the concept. Using three measures of a variable provides a margin of safety: If A is unrelated to B, there is still hope that C will relate to either A or B, and a relationship between any pair helps define their conceptual commonality. Unless measures have known validity, it seems wise to use at least three.

This advice must be accompanied by a caution. There may be a good deal of autonomy or independence among verbal, autonomic, and overt responses [47, 50, 52–55, 64], and the investigator should not be surprised if relationships between physiological, verbal, and expressive measures are weak. Such a case might argue for at least three physiological, three verbal, and three expressive indices to increase the possibility of coherence at each level. In testing for consistency across levels, we would hope to use, at the minimum, at least two interrelated measures at each level.

If the researcher follows this recommendation, her measures may proliferate beyond a number she can manage either conceptually or financially. There are several solutions to this problem. First, if a clear theoretical model exists, it can provide the investigator with a priori ideas of the levels she should measure and often, in addition, with a priori hypotheses about the meaning of specific patterns of the measures; e.g., see the studies comparing strong verbalizers who have weak physiological responses with strong physiological responders who have weak verbal responses [51, 85]. With no clear theoretical guide to choice of levels, the investigator should probably stay within a single level, measuring only overt behavior or verbalization, for example. But she should probably collect her overt behavior (or verbal) data in several different ways, to insure that consistency between measures does not derive solely from commonalities in the method of measurement; e.g., answers based on a seven-point scale to three attitude questions might be in agreement but diverge sharply from coded responses to open-ended attitude questions.

Again, if the patient's medical problem involves a specific organ, such as the heart, it may be of special importance to include measures of cardiac activity along with any other behavioral measures used for concept definition. This will provide needed information on the relationship between variations in the behavioral measures and activity in the organ directly affected by the disease processes.

In order to validate her measures, the investigator may introduce a known factor as a criterion for the interpretation of the other measures. This factor could be either some validated response measure or some independent variable known to have powerful effects on the process of interest. For example, in their study of stress reactions of women in labor, Leventhal, Ellsberry, and Kedar [56] took repeated verbal, postural, and sweat measures as the patient came closer to delivery. Since contractions intensify with increasing dilation over time, any measure showing significant relationships to dilation probably detects changes in intensity of stimulation and is, therefore, probably a valid measure of distress.

This example makes clear how closely the interpretation or validity of a response measure can be tied to environmental variations. Thus, if two out of three measures of distress intercorrelate, but the two do not vary with changes in known environmental stressors – e.g., increased dilation, presence or absence of pain medication [59] – and the third measure does relate to these stressors, it is probable that only the third records distress and that the two that are interrelated measure some other factor. The more environmental stressors to which the third relates, the more plausible is this conclusion. Very persuasive evidence of convergence exists when at least two manipulations different in type produce common changes in the same factor [27]. Together, both types of convergence – correlated responses and common effects from independent manipulations – provide the most persuasive evidence for the interpretation of the concept and the meaning of the response measures.

Drawing Conclusions from Multiple Measures

We have stressed the importance of multiple measures as a means to determine whether or not one is measuring a specific concept. The discussion has focused on the validity of measures and in particular that aspect of validity called construct validity [17]. How realistic is it to expect our measures to show high consistency in defining a concept, and what kinds of conclusions can we draw, for example, if our verbal, expressive, and physiological measures of distress do not interrelate closely?

Not surprisingly, there are a number of resolutions to the problem of inconsistency between measures. Campbell and Fiske [4] argue that a concept is not adequately defined unless several different types of measures give equivalent results, and they add a more stringent requirement: that the measures that define a concept cannot correlate with measures defining other, unrelated concepts. That is, if our verbal and expressive measures of distress converge, but correlate as well with our measures of joy, we may question whether we are measuring distress at all. Indeed, the example suggests that we are measuring level of activation or arousal rather than any particular emotion.

Campbell and Fiske's approach makes many important points for the study of individual differences. For example, Mischel [73] suggests that many of the relationships reported between measures of personality traits and later performance in school or on the job are easily accounted for by the fact that the trait measure and job performance both relate to intelligence; the trait measure thus adds nothing to our understanding of job performance.

This is a good example of discriminant validity; if the trait concept is of value, it should be measurable and its measures should relate to other variables in a way that is different from the relationship found for measures of intelligence.

Is the Campbell and Fiske approach fully applicable to measurement of behavioral processes in the nursing research setting, or do differences in this setting qualify their recommendations? Campbell and Fiske's proposals were designed to handle the phenomena of individual differences, and in that area each measure is supposed to refer to a concept (e.g., trait, ability) that represents a relatively stable underlying determinant of individual differences in behavior. Thus the measures of a concept should be stable over time and correlate only with one another and not with measures of other concepts. However, in the nursing setting, our process model refers to events unstable over time, and the measures of the underlying concepts are likely to fluctuate sharply with fluctuations in the emotional and coping processes involved in adapting to the setting. Convergent validation for these concepts must thus grapple with the fact that multiple measures of a concept may converge only at the precise moment in time when the conceptual process is in operation. Other processes may be in play at other times, and the measures may assess entirely different sets of concepts.

These considerations make clear that it may be difficult to demonstrate convergent validity by a correlational approach unless we are certain that the measures for each person are taken at identical points in the unfolding of the process. For example, suppose we use four measures of distress – efforts to avoid the doctor, verbal report, heart rate, skin conductance – to assess response to a treatment procedure which involves a series of painful events. If we do not measure the behaviors at identical points in the process for each person, the correlations between the autonomic measures and the other responses, when computed across persons, could be relatively low, especially if some people show more rapid adaptation in the autonomic system than in the behavior system.

There are several ways to handle this problem. One alternative is to compute the means for each score at different points in time and to intercorrelate these means; a high r would show that on the average the measures respond similarly over time. An alternative to correlations computed across patients or between means is to take a series of measures on each patient and to compute correlations between the measures separately for each patient. Thus, even if some people show fairly rapid adaptation of their autonomic responses but not of their verbal responses, which would lower a between-subject correlation, their autonomic responses soon after the distressful event will still be high in comparison with the resting level. A correlation between verbal and autonomic acts within a subject could still show high internal consistency.

An important caution must be kept in mind when examining correlations computed within subjects. These correlations are often artificially inflated by the specific features of the situation in which the data are collected. For example, Malmstrom, Opton, and Lazarus [64] reported high intraindividual correlations between measures of galvanic skin response and heart rate in subjects viewing a stress film. They argued that correlations between measures are always higher when computed within subjects rather than between subjects, because correlations computed for scores between subjects are dependent on the people sampled. If the people are highly similar on one or both of the two measures correlated, the correlation tends to be lowered. But they failed to realize that the magnitude of a correlation computed for a person across occasions depends on the sample of the occasions. In the latter case, a small sample of measures that fall into two sharply different classes, painful and non-painful, may yield higher correlations that would be found if the situations varied less or if they varied along many dimensions other than pain.

An interesting problem is encountered in experimental studies when two or three behavioral measures of a concept show similar relationships across treatment conditions but are unrelated to one another when correlations are calculated within treatments [65]; or when two behavioral measures correlate within experimental conditions but do not show the same pattern of change across treatment conditions [58]. We can take two different approaches to these puzzling outcomes.

The first approach is to assume that we are dealing with two *alternative, disjunctive* measures of a single concept. For example when person A was about to be operated on, he showed physiological changes but did not talk about it; B talked a lot about how distressed he felt but showed little physiological reactivity; yet both are equally distressed. We would assume that we need both measures – physiological and verbal report – to detect the common underlying state, as each detects only some proportion of the anxiety or distress [37]. This interpretation is especially reasonable if we have theoretical reasons for expecting the two measures to be disjunctive; that is, if we expect high expressivity actually to lower the autonomic response (e.g., skin conductance), while low expressivity increases it. In this instance it would be wise to compute correlations between measures separately for each person. These correlations could show the inverse relationship between overt and internal expressivity and might do so even if the disjunction held only for some rather than for all patients.

The second approach to the problem posed by the outcome in which treatments affect different indicators for different people is to assume that we are dealing with different processes (or concepts) in each subgroup of patients. Thus we could conclude that patients showing high levels of expressive behavior postsurgically manifest distress type A, while patients having high levels of autonomic response show distress type B. This may seem unparsimonious, and it certainly leads to a more complex model than that which assumes we have alternative measures of a common concept of distress. But there are a number of research areas where complexity has proved closer to truth than simplicity.

For example, in his fascinating review of the dramatic work on arousal, Lacey [46] concludes that we can no longer hope to find *the* best measure of arousal or the best set of measures for this concept. He reasons that there is no such thing as a unitary concept of arousal. The organism's "level of activation" is a composite of several arousal subsystems, including separate systems for cortical, behavioral, and autonomic activity. It is true that under many, if not most, circumstances these systems work cooperatively; we are usually cortically alert when behaviorally active. But there are conditions where one can find a somnolent animal with arousal shown on the electroencephalogram (such as rapid eye movement sleep) and other situations where one can find a behaviorally active animal with a sleep wave electroencephalogram. The concept of arousal is simply less unitary than supposed.

We need a way of determining whether to stick with one concept or move to two. It may be the case that arousal is separable into different components, but does the separation make a difference? Perhaps under most circumstances we can act as if arousal were unitary, knowing full well that at more microscopic levels of analysis it is divisible into component reactions. The mechanism for a decision is both theoretical and pragmatic. If we are dealing with more than one concept, we should be able to make different predictions about the antecedents, consequences, and interactions of each concept. If these predictions are verified, we have more than one concept. If they are not confirmed, or if they are confirmed for observations made exclusively at a more molecular level of theorizing, we can use a unitary concept at the higher level of conceptualization.

In dealing with measures of autonomic and verbal behavior, we would perhaps suggest that concepts be more finely discriminated than such concepts as arousal and stress are. In dealing with response to stress, for example, it seems useful to talk about the more specific attitudes toward the stressor, since these attitudes seem to mediate the complex and differentiable patterns of autonomic activity in what may appear to the outsider as homogeneous stress situations. Graham and his associates [28, 29] present suggestive evidence for the hypothesis that whether a subject feels victimized and helpless or victimized and desirous of striking back determines whether one obtains autonomic response patterns characteristic of illnesses such as hives, hypertension, or Reynaud's disease – a hypothesis of theoretical and pragmatic significance to nursing.

Theory clearly plays a crucial part in untangling the meaning of any data set. Knowledge of the attitude theory of expressive pattern would suggest taking various measures of attitude in addition to psychophysiological measures and verbal measures of discomfort and distress. The theory points to the measures to be taken and to the analyses to be performed.

Ongoing research continually clarifies our concepts. In fact, it may be that we will find such novel and complex relationships between our measures of distress or anxiety that we will invent entirely new concepts reflecting the coherence of these operational dimensions. Research functions to replace old concepts with new, but only when a careful examination of empirical findings requires the change. In this way our concepts become even better representations of our hypothetical "reality."

OBSERVATION

Once the investigator has defined her concept in terms of appropriate measures, she must choose relevant methods of *observation.* At the conceptual stage we sought to exclude inappropriate measures from our definition of concept, to reduce the likelihood that the measures actually defined some other concept than the one under study. Similarly, at the observing stage, we seek to exclude contamination from our recording of the measures, again, to reduce the chance that our observation records something other than the concept under study. We shall consider this issue of validity first in general terms, more specifically as it relates to types, timing, and condition of observation, and most specifically as it relates to observation of verbal behavior.

Internal and External Validity

Problems of recording behavior in any study design can be viewed in terms of the internal and external validity of the findings [15]. The question of internal validity asks whether we have the conditions and measures needed to define a particular concept and distinguish it from other potentially confounding concepts. External validity refers to generalizability of the findings and raises questions about the applicability of the findings to other settings; for example, whether or not the patient population is typical or the illnesses studied usual. It is extremely important to protect the internal validity of all experiments; without it one cannot draw conclusions about the processes involved in the behavior.

Traditionally, the applied researcher has been more concerned with external than internal validity. But as Leventhal [55] has stressed elsewhere, one cannot necessarily expect to generalize directly from experimental results to the practice setting. Indeed, it may prove disastrous to design studies and methods to maximize external generalization. A good experiment allows one to tease out precisely how specific factors affect one or another response measure; it has high internal validity. One may be tempted to allow several factors to vary together to enhance external validity, i.e., to do "realistic" experiments. But confounding of variables and of causal links is a necessary outcome of experiments that compare global and different nursing practices, since each practice consists of many parts. The confounded study may be more externally valid and be generalizable immediately to practice, but it does not tell us which factors in the treatments relate to the difference obtained.

This state of affairs is potentially more serious than it may seem. First, many of the components of the preferred practice may be costly, inefficient, and unnecessary for its success. Second, a change in a component of one of the less successful treatments may make it superior to all others. Third, the success of one practice over others may depend on contextual factors which, if changed, would completely alter the study outcome. For example, in decades when patients are passive and accepting, authoritarian practices might prove more effective than those that give the patient control over his situation. But in an era when patients have decided to be self-controlling, the opposite may be true. Since no one knows what the future may bring, it seems wise to proceed in the slower, more careful way to discover the role of particular variables and their interactions with environmental or contextual factors, in short, to proceed theoretically and with high internal validity.

As one consequence of this position, the nurse-researcher may have to think of more than one type of research. Carefully designed studies high in internal validity would be important to establish a model of the behavioral processes involved in patient care. The investigator would then generalize this theory to other complex practice settings. This second phase might involve multivariate research, with instruments to measure and interrelate different process and outcome variables in the most complex practice setting. This research could generate knowledge of the applicability of the model to practice and suggest other specific studies of context factors and previously unsuspected interactions. The points we will raise about data collection and analysis would apply to both types of research as well as to studies falling between these extremes.

Types of Observers

HUMAN OBSERVERS

One simple way to collect data is to have an experimenter present to record the behavior, which can be of several types: things the patient says – attitudes, information, values, moods (verbal measures); things he does – sleeps, reads, calls nurses, walks around (instrumental or expressive activity); or changes in his body (physiological activity). In all cases, the experimenter records behavior as it occurs. While most straightforward, this approach presents several problems.

The Patient's Awareness of the Recording Process. When a patient is directly observed, he nearly always senses it. Observation itself may cause him to alter his behavior. Thus a sick person may feel it his duty to look and act sick when there are observers in the environment, or he may try to obtain attention and care from the medical staff by acting sick. In either case, the patient's activity strengthens his distress signals on verbal, expressive, and autonomic levels of response. This does not mean that the responses under observation do not reflect pain or discomfort. It merely implies that the measures, and perhaps the intensity of discomfort itself, are influenced by the opportunity to communicate and are partly independent of the illness or healing process.

On the other hand, observational devices may minimize discomfort. They may reassure the patient, convincing him that he is under skilled surveillance, or they may simply interest or distract him. Any of these influences can decrease scores on discomfort responses as well as the discomfort itself, and any such influence obviously affects both the internal and external validity of the study.

The Experimenter's Awareness of the Recording Process. A patient's reactions can be affected by the experimenter's knowledge as well as by his own. Thus the experimenter's knowledge or expectations about how the subject will behave may create "demand characteristics" [74] or bias the patient's behavior in other more subtle ways [77]. Orne [74] used the term *demand characteristic* to describe the fact that subjects in experiments are much more likely to follow the orders of the authoritarian experimenter than similar orders given in nonexperimental settings. More subtle biases result when the experimenter conveys clues to the patient about his expected behavior. For example, a nurse giving back rubs or relaxation treatment may tell the patient by tone of voice or other subtle cues that she expects him to report less distress. The patient, to show his appreciation of the nurse's efforts, to be a good subject, or to keep her from feeling she has failed, may distort his report or control his expression so that he appears to feel less distress than before. On the other hand, while engaging in the nursing procedures for a control subject, the nurse may unwittingly influence the patient to report that he is uncomfortable. The distress measures and the comparisons between the conditions may have little or nothing to do with the nursing practice; the comparison is not internally valid and cannot be generalized.

At times, however, demand characteristics may be a part of an experimental manipulation. For example, if the nurse tells the patient that she hopes to reduce his distress with a back rub, and the patient afterward not only shows less distress but feels less, then the manipulation is successful. The problem is to distinguish the "real" change in distress from a false effect, created when the patient misrepresents his internal state. The experimenter may even test for the importance of the verbalization of expectations ("This is to make you feel better.") by giving the back rub without and with the remark. The experimenter may also wish to select a behavioral measure that is not easily biased; e.g., if the nurse's goal is to help a patient stop smoking, and she tells him this, she would be wise to measure actual smoking behavior and not rely on a verbal report.

Like the nurse or manipulator of the experimental condition, the observer or recorder can be a source of cues or demands to the patient which will bias experimental findings. The cues of both manipulator and observer usually arise out of their *knowledge of the hypothesis* under test, their expectations of the outcome, and by knowledge of the condition (experimental or control) to which the patient is assigned. Bias through the observer can be eliminated if she is ignorant of the study hypothesis and of the contrasting experimental or control conditions, or kept ignorant (blind) to the condition to which a particular subject has been assigned.

It is obviously easier to keep the observer blind when her recording is subsequent to the experimental manipulation. But if she must also rate the manipulation, it is impossible to keep her unbiased; in this instance the researcher should consider separate observers for each task [39].

Bias through the manipulator is harder to eliminate, because it is more difficult to keep her ignorant of the experimental condition. In the laboratory, ignorance can be maintained if the experimenter does not actually deliver the instructions that differentiate experimental groups. For example, it is a common practice to run several experimental conditions simultaneously with the differential instructions conveyed through printed or tape-recorded messages. It is more difficult to use such devices for a nursing manipulation. When a blind procedure cannot be followed, it may be possible to build careful checks on the independent variables into the research. For example, films and tape recordings of the experimental manipulations allow rating of experimenter performance on a variety of factors [57]; or transcribed nurse-patient interactions may be read by a competent, disinterested person and judged against a set of criteria describing varied nursing approaches [22].

The Observer as a Condition. We have dealt with the ways in which the observer's and experimenter's knowledge of both hypotheses and assignment to experimental conditions biases the experiment. It should be added, however, that the very act of studying a phenomenon may create or exaggerate differences between experimental treatments. For example, an observer may not know the hypothesis of the experiment or the experimental group of the subject, yet she may increase the reactivity of all subjects in the study by her mere presence and eagerness to make observations. Raising the reactivity level of the patients can strengthen the processes that are active in both experimental and control patients. For example, if patients in a control group are slightly anxious and upset while patients in an experimental nursing group are slightly interested in the nursing care they are receiving, adding to the arousal level of both groups will strengthen each of these processes and make the control group appear more anxious and the experimental group more interested or involved with their care. There is a good deal of evidence that the mere presence of an observer can have a drive or multiplying effect [95]. In this instance merely introducing an unbiased observer has reduced the external validity of the experimental results; i.e., the multiplying effect will make for a bigger difference between conditions than would appear in the usual practice setting when no observer is present. To deal with this problem, one might minimize the obtrusiveness of the observation or allow extra time for patients to adapt to it. One might also estimate the observer effect by making unobtrusive observations on another sample.[2]

MECHANICAL OBSERVERS

To eliminate biases resulting from the presence of a human observer, investigators frequently use mechanical recording devices. Although such devices seem impartial and less likely to introduce demands or bias, they are no panacea. If he can see the mechanical recorder, the patient knows he is being observed and may try to guess what response is wanted. Preprogramming the recorder may help to eliminate differential cues to the experimental conditions, both to the patient and to people scoring the behavioral record. But if the recorder is operated by a person, it can still introduce biases. For example, in recording facial expressions in interactions, a human operator may selectively record or may use the equipment differently in different experimental conditions, thereby providing cues and altering the patient's behavior.

INDIRECT OBSERVATION

Whether mechanical or human, direct observation can be costly as well as reactive (i.e., productive of false differences). A less costly and less reactive approach to data collection is an indirect one: the use of environmental "deposits," that is, physical effects or other records left by the patient's behavior. In their book *Unobtrusive Measures,* Webb and colleagues [90] discuss a number of such indirect measures, many of which are available in the hospital setting. For example, the dosage of analgesics and the frequency of administration could serve as a measure of distress, with possible confounding factors such as the physician's prescription held constant. The condition of a patient's bedding also could provide cues to his psychological state; creased and stained sheets reflect excessive restlessness and sweating. The hospital charts provide data on drugs taken, food eaten, time asleep, vomiting, and length of hospital stay. No one of these is likely to be definitive, but each could provide useful supplementary data. Moreover, the resourceful investigator in a favorable setting can solicit and obtain cooperation to improve the quality of these measures. For example, if pain medication is given by rigidly defined schedules that depend on the type of surgery, or body weight, or both, the use of medication would not indicate distress. But if the rules for prescription are reworked so as to specify minimum and maximum dosages, variation in usage could then reflect the individual needs of the patient; and differences between patients would probably relate to their psychological states.

A clear implication of the discussion of experimenter and observer effects is that so-called psychological factors have an important effect on pain and distress. This effect complicates all our observations, whether indirect, mechanical, or human. The clinical literature offers abundant examples of such influence. Beecher [11] draws a clear distinction between pain and the reaction to pain; the former is a sensory signal, and the latter is primarily an emotional response. Other investigators have also made this distinction [69, 70]. Beecher indicates that the reaction component, which includes important and extensive changes in verbalization, gestures, and visceral activity, is highly variable and susceptible to a wide variety of influences. Thus soldiers with extensive wounds often report no pain because such a report will remove them from battle [10].

Barbiturates and other "tranquilizing" or emotion-reducing drugs are more appropriate than morphine in pain treatment if pain is high because of emotional reactivity. Because the reaction component is sensitive to a wide range of social and environmental variables, the investigator, like the clinician, must take it into account in the design of his studies and data collection procedures. This is not cause for despair; it is a challenge. The investigator-practitioner seeks to understand which factors influence behavior, to develop a theory or model of the process, and to devise ways of bringing these variables under control.

Ethical Considerations. To minimize false effects, it might seem desirable to keep the patient unaware of the recording process. This is something all too easily achieved in this electronic age, but deceiving or not informing the patient raises serious ethical questions. We feel that the patient should be informed of his participation. But clearly many studies could not proceed if the patient knew their purposes in detail. Such knowledge could make him self-conscious or motivate him to act in accord with or against the experimenter's hypothesis. However, there are intermediate levels of information, which allow the patient the freedom to participate yet do not reveal the exact nature of the hypotheses or observations being made.

For example, in a study now nearing completion, Leventhal, Ellsberry, and Kedar [56] made videotapes, palmar sweat records, and verbal response recordings of women during labor. In all cases, the women had consented prior to their participation in the study, and all knew what types of measures were to be obtained. This knowledge reduced the novelty of the data-collection devices and even seemed to minimize their effects on behavior. But the patients did not know the exact purpose of the study, i.e., what the investigators were looking for, nor did they know when the television cameras were actually operating. Clearly, each study poses unique problems, but *intelligent and judicious decisions must safeguard both the patient and the validity of experimental findings.*

Equal emphasis needs to be put on safeguarding the patient's welfare and the validity of research. The practitioner often shows bias toward the immediate welfare of the patient; the practitioner may feel the experimenter callous and indifferent when she withholds a potentially beneficial treatment or uses a treatment that may be emotionally distressing. But there is an ethics to research, and the practitioner who is not a researcher often fails to perceive the harm that can come from poorly controlled studies. Treatment techniques resulting from such poorly structured studies may be used for decades at great expense and harm to patients, and the belief that a valid treatment already exists may inhibit the quest for more efficient, effective, and humane procedures.

There is no reason why thousands of women should suffer the discomfort and joylessness of one or another form of procedure for delivering babies because some supposedly concerned medical professionals refuse to allow a comparison of traditional procedures with so-called natural childbirth methods. Similarly, there is no reason why a small band of enthusiastic and dedicated mothers should impose natural childbirth methods on thousands of subsequent patients who are less enthusiastic and less dedicated if the efficacy of the procedures depends on the enthusiasm of the participants. In short, ethical questions appear whenever we treat without understanding the basis of our treatment. Understanding comes only through careful theoretical and empirical work.

Training Observers

Science is a public enterprise, in the sense that any trained individual, in the same place, at the same time, with the same instruments, subjects, and conditions should observe the same phenomena. Belief in the "reality" of a behavioral event substantially increases when different observers and experimenters obtain identical results. Replication with a change in experimenters helps insure that the result is independent of any particular individual's action or subjective expectation.

However replication of results with new experimenters and observers does not insure scientific validity, for sometimes whole sets of experimenters and observers share similar biases and produce confounded and invalid observations. How, then, should we train observers? Commonly, we try to eliminate bias by providing all observers identical information about their tasks and identical practice and experience performing them. Yet it may be worthwhile to vary the training (or bias) for different observers. If observers with varied training produce identical results, confidence that effects are independent of the observer's beliefs and expectations is increased. Varied training is absolutely necessary when one studies the effects of observer expectations on behavioral recording.

A number of minor but important features must be considered in all observer training. First, the observer must be made familiar with the experimental setting and the recording instrument, whether questionnaire, content analysis scheme, free behavior recording sheet, or mechanical device. When the observer is familiar with her tools, she is at ease and functions more reliably. Although experimenters strive for observer reliability early in training, they often overlook the problem of subtle changes that occur in later stages of data collection. As the members of a study team learn and then overlearn their tasks, they may begin to short-circuit procedures or otherwise alter their behavior and bias their findings. Comparison between observers throughout the duration of a study helps insure stability in the recording instrument, as will checking them against a constant recorder.

Coding their data on women's responses to stress of labor, Leventhal, Ellsberry, and Kedar [56] held daily "tuning sessions." Coders worked on a common case, checked themselves for agreement, discussed shifts in code meaning, and only then proceeded to code. Highly specific coding categories helped, since they required a minimum of inference; coders recorded the occurrence of specific movements within brief time intervals (fifteen-second periods) and did not rate intentions or goals. Finally, though each record of behavior, in this case a six-minute videotape, was scored on several codes, each coder worked on only one code at a time. This reduced the possibility of confusion and sharply increased accuracy and intercoder agreement.

Many other techniques can serve to enhance observer accuracy. For example, Heyns and Zander [35] convinced their coders of the need for precise categories by having them attempt to rate behavior without the help of a coding system. Occurring when they were naive, this experience led raters to understand the wide range of responses that could be coded and helped convince them of the need for precise categories and careful adherence to publicly understandable rules. For a more detailed discussion of observer training, the reader should examine Weick's [91] excellent chapter in the *Handbook of Social Psychology.*

Time of Observation

When should measurements be taken? To answer this question it may be useful to construct a contrast between two extreme situations: (1) the created process and (2) the active or ongoing process. The former process is introduced or created by the experimenter; the latter is present and active prior to experimenter intervention. Most laboratory experiments introduce a stimulus into the subject's life space and create the process they then study. Choosing the time of behavioral observation is simplified, as the interesting behavioral consequences follow the manipulation. However, intuition and extensive pretesting must guide the researcher in selecting the optimal moments for both manipulation and measurement. Moreover, some processes require measures at more than one point in time. For example, members of our research group compared the effects of two motives, emotional and rational appraisal of danger, on smoking reduction [60, 76] and tetanus inoculation [42].

Comparing the effects of these two motives on later behavior, we noted that one was effective at one time and the other was more effective later. Because fear is a momentary emotional response, its motivating effect, whether positive in inhibiting smoking or negative in inhibiting tetanus inoculation, usually showed only immediately after the motive was aroused by a communication. The danger motive, on the other hand, produced effects that persisted for weeks or even months.

Unlike a laboratory investigator, the clinical researcher may have to alter an already active process; a nurse usually does not try to cause distress but rather to intervene at an appropriate time to reduce it. The nurse does not have the problems of the laboratory experimenter who needs to develop an authentic situation to produce a tolerable though noticeable level of distress. While "reality-produced" distress presents advantages over the laboratory variety, the experimenter still faces the problem that distress is not equally available for reduction or observation at all times during hospitalization. For example, when the experimenter studies the best nursing procedure for reducing anxiety during hospital admissions, she should know when distress is at its height and how rapidly it changes without treatment. If distress and anxiety are highest immediately on admission, manipulations and measures should be taken at that point. On the other hand, if the patients are children, distress and anxiety may be delayed, as it may take time for them to become fully aware of their isolation from parents and everyday surroundings. Moreover, different intervention techniques may be successful at different points in the process.

Since the optimal time for observation is hard to choose, particularly in the "real-world" setting, some researchers resort to continuous recording. Unfortunately, data then become excessive, and the investigator may face an impossible task of classification and abstraction. Time sampling may help her out of this dilemma. Observations of different lengths and at varying intervals can provide most of the information found in continual recordings. Timing and duration of observations depend, however, on knowledge of the process – whether it is acute in onset, cumulative in intensity, random in appearance, or cyclical. The well-designed schedule detects the response to experimental conditions and avoids the accumulation of excessive data.

Missing Observations

Missing observations occur in most field studies, and techniques exist for generating data in such cases [83]. It may seem extremely arbitrary to "make up" data, but the procedure can be justified because certain methods of data analysis (e.g., comparisons of a series of post-treatment scores for several groups of patients, covarying pretreatment scores on income, knowledge, intelligence) require equal numbers of observations in each cell of the experiment. Thus, if one observation is lacking for several patients, each on different days, one must either throw out the cases or generate data. Both the costs and the risks of bias can be greater in keeping only those cases that could be continually observed.

It is also important to see if the missing instances present a systematic source of bias. For example, people often refuse to participate or be observed in an experimental setting. More refusals in one experimental group than in another may produce a sampling bias. Bias may also occur when more subjects in one group than another see through elaborate deceptions and are omitted. One group may then contain higher proportions of gullible or suggestible subjects. Equal loss, however, is no assurance of unbiased samples. We can never know if the same experimental effects hold for those who refuse as well as for those who volunteer for an experiment. Moreover, when different instructions are used in different experimental conditions, it is never certain that refusals occur for the same reason in each condition. Thus we may lose different types of patients in each condition.

Data may also be missing because of failure to question all respondents. An interview may be written so that some questions are asked only if one has given particular answers to earlier questions or if one has particular characteristics. For example, mothers having their first child may be asked a different selection of questions than mothers having a second or third. While these differences between respondents may make certain questions inapplicable, the investigator will find that she can often reword a question so that it will apply to all individuals in the sample. By obtaining data on all members of the sample she will be able to make comparisons between subgroups that will help her to interpret the meaning of the responses.

Verbal Behavior

As previously mentioned, some scientists may assume that only physiological data or data about the patients' physical activities warrant objective scientific treatment. Consequently, they may regard verbal behavior – what patients say as opposed to what they or their bodies do – as subjective and inadequate for scientific treatment. Other investigators emphatically disagree. Kaplan [41] illustrates the value of speech and retells a fable about the arrival of an object from outer space. Physicists and astronomers perform a variety of tests to determine the object's identity, composition, and structure. Their efforts fail to penetrate its mystery. Finally, a psychologist arrives, approaches the object and asks, "What's your name?" The object replies, "Ralph." While the answer failed to provide a complete solution to the problem, it suggested more than any other datum.

In all behavioral research, one must measure relevant behavior, those crucial responses that provide the most valid indices of our concepts. Certain things can most easily be discovered through words, and other things cannot be discovered in any other way; e.g., subjective events like the patients' feelings, attitudes, moods, and experiences of pain. Moreover, the professionals who care for the patient rely heavily on his own report of his state; and when researchers utilize measures of the same kind as those used in practice, they not only facilitate the use of their findings in the practice setting, but insure that the practitioner can actually obtain data relevant to the processes under investigation. Here, research serves to verify a hypothesis and a method of data collection used by both practitioner and researcher.

Some subjective events, such as attitudes and values, can endure a long time, while others, such as moods, can fluctuate rapidly. Duration is no guide to importance, since a rapidly changing emotion may be as important to the patient's welfare as a more slowly changing belief. We must ask whether or not the process in question is relevant to our research interests. If we decide that it is, we must then deal with whatever measurement problems it presents.

Words can reflect underlying processes as surely as pulse rate or any other datum that appears more clearly tied to physical happenings. Verbal behavior *is* behavior. It "exists," and it can be recorded objectively, classified, counted, and quantified. As with any other kind of behavior, the real problem is how to measure it in reliable and valid ways.

DATA COLLECTION

Verbal behavior can be sampled by direct questioning or by recording spontaneous productions. Questioning includes interviews, questionnaires, and tests (e.g., of information, personality) and ranges from highly structured sessions in which a list of questions is used to casual conversations or even group discussions. In gathering *spontaneous* verbalization, the researcher does not interact with the patient, but in either spontaneous or structured conversation she sorts out and categorizes what she hears.

Many experiments combine direct questioning and spontaneous recording. For example, seeking distress measures for patients in labor, we might record such spontaneous verbalizations as the number of "ouches," "oohs," and screams and other verbal signs of discomfort. But if some apparently distressed women who do not scream are discovered, a direct interview will be needed to assess whether they inhibit spontaneous verbalization and therefore do not feel distress or use other verbal reactions to describe their feelings. Much research combines the two methods, and from this point on the discussion pertains to both.

WORDS AND "REALITY"

While we have stressed the reality of processes behind verbal behavior, it is naive to assume that words correspond one to one with these processes. Sometimes people cannot report processes because they are not wholly conscious of them. Deliberately or not, people sometimes say what they think others want to hear. Sometimes people simply lie. Generally, if we ask a patient for explanations of his behavior, he will probably report the most proximate causes, or what he believes are socially desirable reasons for his action [19]. Motives of behavior are the investigator's or nurse's concepts and not necessarily the patient's concepts. The patient can tell you that he called the nurse and what he wanted to ask her, but this doesn't mean that he can describe the dependency motive or the anxiety that led him to seek contact. The patient can tell you that he is frightened, bored, fatigued, or angry, and give you his perception of the causes of his feelings. But this does not mean that he has accurately identified the cause of his feelings and that if the cause is clarified his feelings may abruptly change. There is absolutely no reason to believe that the patient can directly report on the factors that mediate his behavior. Indeed, this is what research seeks to understand, and these processes are inferred from systematic alterations in behavior caused by a changing environment (which includes body chemistry and structure).

Although questions do not provide a direct way of detecting determinants of behavior, the verbal report can still tell us a great deal about the patient who gives it. Like overt, or autonomic behavior, the verbal report gives data. The nurse construes the meaning of the verbal report in the context of a coding system and of an experiment where she can observe relationships between systematically manipulated environmental events and the frequency of responses in specific code categories.

The researcher must learn which statements may be taken at face value and which may not be. But anyone who believes that verbal behavior per se is subjective and unreliable should examine the research literature in perception. When situations are properly structured, a human being can detect minute amounts of photic or auditory stimulation, and discriminate between hundreds of colors and tones, and can express these discriminations verbally. The accuracy of these verbal reports derives in large part from the stimulus setting. Typically, the subject simultaneously compares two stimuli and is asked to state, even if he must guess, which of the two is, for example, brighter, louder, or redder. Even when the subject believes that he cannot make these judgments, he will accurately discriminate very small differences [18, 25]. People can discriminate far less when they judge stimuli one at a time rather than comparing two stimuli to one another [72]. However, researcher ingenuity can improve even single stimulus judgments [84] and experiments suggest that subjects can utilize even a 20-point rating scale for some judgments [26]. Researchers can apply techniques from these perception studies to more complex verbal judgments such as those for pain [10, 32] and emotional distress [40].

In general, verbal behavior is most reliable when it reports a person's immediate experience. If we keep this in mind along with the points to be mentioned, we can readily design questions to elicit reliable and valid verbal reports.

GOAL OF THE QUESTION

Questions may seek data on a person's attitudes, values, feelings, moods, emotions, information and knowledge, and behavior. To know one of these is not necessarily to know about another; people's attitudes and behavior, knowledge, and feelings are not necessarily congruent. For example, if we study the emotional stress induced by upcoming surgery, our questions should get at feelings and not just knowledge of surgery. Similarly, a patient's general attitude toward nurses, and knowledge about their work, is not equivalent to his feelings about the nursing care he is receiving! The researcher must decide precisely what she wishes to measure and then develop operational equivalents of her concepts; i.e., questions which tap only these experiences and actions. And if she wants meaningful data, she will ask one thing at a time; what the patient feels (Do you feel pain? Do you feel nausea?), where he feels it, how long it lasts, etc. Questions about two or more states at a time defy clear response and produce obscure data.

FORM OF THE QUESTION

Once we have defined the goal of the question, we must define its form. Closed questions specify response possibilities a priori. The subject marks his response on a scale, or chooses from a fixed set of answers, or agrees or disagrees with a statement. Open questions, on the other hand, do not directly suggest any answers to the subject; the subject supplies his own, which may range from a simple "yes" or "no" to a long rambling story.

Both open and closed questions present advantages and disadvantages. Compared to closed questions, open questions avoid putting words in a subject's mouth. His response reflects the degree to which an issue is *truly salient for him.* Specifically, a closed question might ask a patient to agree or disagree with the statement, "Doctors should inform their patients of the purpose of all treatments." We would categorize a patient who agrees with this statement as one who "feels it is important to know the purpose of treatments." But this may not be true, and this is the main drawback of the closed question. Though the patient agreed when he encountered the question, he may never have thought about it if left to himself. Of course, his agreement might predict how he would react when and if he were treated and not given information.

The open question has its drawbacks, too. Responses are often difficult to code; there are problems in determining the equivalence of meaning of different statements and difficulties in developing codes that preserve the differentiations in the original material in a way that is useful for analysis. Some patients also find it hard to stick to the point, and much material may be irrelevant. Evidence exists that demand characteristics (e.g., the interviewer's apparent social class, dress, manner; interview context) and other sources of bias affect open as well as closed responses [23, pp. 338–340; 63, pp. 475–479]. Patients withhold some answers and tailor others to felt demand. Thus even open questions may not indicate salient issues. But when we just begin to explore a domain, open questions best enable us to discover which issues are important, which responses most likely, and which mode of approach is most likely to generate relevant answers. Patients' answers may provide clues to items and relationships not thought of, and at this early stage one can follow them up without worrying about comparability and coding.

In the later stages of research, the properly constructed, well-pretested closed question is the better tool. It is readily codable, answers are comparable, and it insures that we have tapped the relevant dimensions. Combinations of closed and open questions are also useful. For example, we might arrive at a form in which we first ask subjects, "Have you ever thought about whether a doctor should inform patients about the purpose of treatments?" One could then ask patients how they feel about the statement, "Doctors should inform their patients of the purposes of all treatments," and ask them to indicate whether they agree strongly or mildly, or are indifferent, or disagree mildly or strongly. Here the open question allows us to assess the patient's present level of interest and concern with the issue, and the following closed questions allow for an easily codable and directly comparable response. The open question identifies idiosyncratic views and also provides an opportunity for the subject to consider the issue before giving a scaled answer.

PRETESTING

The movement from open to closed questions should take place in a program of thorough pretesting. In pretesting, we discover areas of salience and the best ways of tapping them. Pretesting also demonstrates the understandability of our questions. Since style, vocabulary, and phrasing all affect the answers given to questions, the pretest should also examine these [23, pp. 342–350; 63, pp. 455–459]. Another of the important tasks in pretesting is simply to look at the responses obtained to see whether or not they tell us about relevant processes. Obscure and irrelevant answers suggest the need to redefine questions; and sometimes they remind us that we cannot learn everything through questions, especially with limited samples or in special settings, and they may suggest a new research tack altogether.

CODES FOR CONTENT ANALYSIS

Content analysis is a topic far too extensive for detailed coverage here. The reader might examine a recent treatment by Holsti and his collaborators [36]. But the following points are worth making here.

First, content analysis cannot readily proceed without a theoretical conception to guide the formulation of categories and coding rules. To develop a coding system, one states rules for the classification of responses and develops specific examples of the application of rules to samples of verbal behavior. The very same verbal contents can be examined and coded for a variety of purposes. Thus, in coding the interaction between patient and nurse, the investigator needs to consider, for example, whether her goal is to make inferences about the communicator (the patient) or to describe the patient's verbalizations as stimuli for the nurse. She may also want to develop a code system to detect the influence of contextual factors (e.g., nursing task, presence or absence of doctor, family member) on the verbalizations of patient and nurse. Each goal, detecting the influence of the communicator, recipient, and/or setting, shapes the codes in particular ways.

The coding system is also tied to the experimental design; the same questions we have raised about behavioral observations in general apply with equal force to a coding system. Thus the investigator should raise questions about how coded data can and should relate to independent variables in her experimental design. She will test variations in the frequency over time of code categories: settings, sources, recipients, tasks, nursing procedures, style of interpersonal contact, types of information given the patient before hospitalization or at admission or during medical procedures, and so on. She tests the validity of the category, i.e., whether or not a particular rule really detects evidence for a specific process and examines the relationship of the category to other response measures and to various independent or treatment factors.

McClelland and Atkinson's [66] development of a "need for achievement" measure presents a striking example of the development of a coding system. The investigators have developed a complex rule book to score stories told about pictures from the thematic apperception test (TAT). The rules allow the codes to decide whether or not a story can be scored for need achievement (that is, it shows competition with others or competition with standards of excellence). If the story meets this criterion, the strength of the need can be scored by coding factors such as statements regarding specific acts to attain goals and regarding barriers to achievement [3]. The system is detailed and possesses adequate reliability and validity. For example, studies have shown that situational conditions can increase and decrease thematic content that is achievement-related [4]; that individuals who score high on the test differ from low scorers in willingness to take risks (high achievers take moderate risks), effort expended in the absence of monetary rewards (high achievers work harder), and preference for working at tasks that are of little, moderate, or great difficulty (high achievers prefer moderately difficult tasks) [5]. Once again, the relationships between code behavior and subsequent behavior validate the meaning of the measure. Several investigators [12, 34, 92] have reviewed the research that has been done on achievement-related responses.

ANALYSIS

Quantification of Data

In all studies the investigator attempts to measure particular events and to compare the measurements for different experimental conditions or to see how different measures relate to one another within the same group of people. Many people feel that a good measure must have the properties of a ratio scale. Ratio scales, such as measures of distance and weight, are highly refined conceptually. They have specific units, which can vary in number from zero to infinity. They allow us to order quantities, to compare differences between one pair of measures and another, and even to say how many times larger one measure is than another. However, many attributes have been meaningfully measured with far less elegant scales. Measurement and research are possible even though the scales used fall far short of ratio measurement.

SCALES

Category Scales. The first step in measurement is to define what is being measured. This definition specifies a particular behavioral response. The specification of the response unit is the most crucial and basic condition for measurement. Once the unit has been specified (usually by defining its beginning and end), measurement proceeds simply and enumerates the frequency of occurrence of the response during some time interval. For example, an investigator might define forehead contractions as signs of distress [59] and count the frequency with which these responses appear within a five-minute period. Thus the specification of a category, and the enumeration of instances within it, form the most primitive type of measurement and the simplest expression of a theoretical concept.

Ordinal, Interval, and Ratio Scales. After categorizing observations, the investigator may attempt to place them in some order of magnitude. The more precisely she can do this the more information she obtains from her measurements. The next order of precision is the ordinal scale. Here, she simply ranks the observations from largest to smallest. Imagine 30 patients who have participated in a study of stress reduction, 15 in an experimental and 15 in a control group. A category scale shows us who did and who did not receive a score, and might show us that most patients, regardless of group, exhibited some signs of distress. But if we rank the patients from most to least stressed, we might see that the experimental group had substantially lower ranks than the control.

Interval scales are still more precise. They tell how much stress each person showed and how far apart the subjects were (in terms of a fixed amount) from one another. The ratio scale adds a true zero point to the equal size interval, so that we can express two magnitudes as a ratio of their respective distances from zero. Thus the ratio scale permits all the statements made with all the other scales: that A is distressed and B is not (categorical scale); that A's distress is greater than B's, and B's is greater than C's (ordinal scale); that the interval *a* to *c* is equal to the sum of the intervals within it [*a* to *b* + (*b* to *c*) = (*a* to *c*) interval scale]. Finally, it allows us to state that B's distress is, for example, twice, one half, or one third as much as A's.

Implications of Scales. While measurement and research may begin with simple scales and few assumptions, the serious investigator and the concerned practitioner press toward increasingly precise quantification, which permits more elegant statements of theory and more exact tests of theoretically derived hypotheses, as the following example illustrates:

An investigator who says that twice as much distress is reduced by nursing method A than by method B assumes she has a ratio scale of distress; that she has met the assumption of equal scale units and a true zero point. In categorical form, her distress measure permits her only to say that the conditions differ in the amount of stress reduced. Ratio quantification would permit more precision and elegance in theory and statement and could have important pragmatic consequences.

Analysis of Observations

To present results and draw conclusions from experimental findings, data must be summarized and estimates made of the statistical significance of the results. If a nurse conducts a study comparing two types of nursing practice, each with 100 patients, and observes each patient five times, she produces 1000 scores. To understand 1000 separate scores is impossible. Her first task is to reduce the scores to some meaningful form, using descriptive devices such as means, percentages, charts, and graphs. Next, she must test the hypothesis about the differences between experimental treatments or the associations between pairs of variables. Here, of course, inferential statistical analysis enters.

Many excellent volumes review the techniques for comparing experimental treatments and correlating sets of variables [20, 33, 68, 82, 88], and it is unnecessary to discuss these in detail here. But a few points do merit emphasis within this context.

VISUAL EXAMINATION

If one were to develop a fantasy of the idealized experiment in this age of technology, the experimenter would have no contact with her subject and see nothing but the final data. Behavior would be recorded automatically and fed to a computer whose output would yield means and probability statements. While this would minimize the work of the experimenter, it would not necessarily maximize the quality of her research. Even today, data merit visual examination. The computer does not hinder such examination since it can print out distributions.

What can visual examination yield? First, it can quickly reveal whether scores within the experimenter's conditions sharply depart from the assumptions behind different statistical tests. For example, parametric tests assume that the underlying distributions and the data are normally distributed. But frequency distributions seldom reveal perfect bell-shaped curves. Fortunately, significance testing procedures, such as the analysis of variance, are reasonably robust, so that their accuracy in estimating the reliability of differences does not seriously diminish even with considerable departures from normality.

Of course, if an investigator examines her distributions separately for each of her experimental treatments and sees that some are bimodal, others flat, some clustered around one or two scale points of the mean, and others spread out nine or ten points, she may suspect that the analysis of variance may not be appropriate for her data and test for this [33, p. 380]. Of equal importance, however, her examination may reveal features of the data that would otherwise escape notice. Bimodal distributions within an experimental treatment, or extreme variability within the experimental as compared with the control treatment, could mean that the treatment works only for some patients; factors such as differences in age, sex, education, or extent of disease may be altering the benefit a patient receives from the treatment. The data can then be examined in detail for such associations. Extreme differences in variance across groups might also suggest problems with unequal scale units, and the data could then be transformed to logarithms or some other unit that minimizes the problem. In dealing with these problems, the investigator would have to decide whether she was confronting the influence of an uncontrolled variable, such as age, or the influence of instability in metric unit induced by factors such as unusually high scores on the dependent variable (e.g., heart rate, muscle tension) in one or more of the conditions [47–49].

One danger in the visual examination of data and the finding of unexpected effects due to uncontrolled factors is overtesting the data. Summed and split often enough, any data set produces significant findings, and we may wind up attending to chance effects. Because of this, the results of such internal analysis are credible only if they fit prestated hypotheses or patterns in previously published research or are replicated in later research.

Data collected in a time series can be usefully examined for the distribution of each individual's scores. For example, suppose that scores are recorded for 30 patients at five points in time. Most investigators present a group curve for the five measures. But is the group curve indicative of individual performance? It may show a consistent increase in distress over time, while the individual curves reveal that some patients arrive with very high distress scores that show no gain, while in other patients, scores rise gradually or very late in the experimental sequence. Possibly, patients whose distress is a response to the setting need different techniques for distress alleviation than those with continually elevated scores.

The researcher can also profitably examine her data through graphs or other pictorial devices. Bar graphs and other devices can instantly reveal systematic effects and "speak" more clearly than a table of mean values.

Visual examination proves especially important when comparing more than two experimental conditions. Figure 5-1 presents mock findings of distress for four experimental groups based on the combination of two nursing variables: physical contact and verbal exploration. Each example shows verbalization with contact more effective than either treatment alone. However, the pattern differs greatly in each case. For *a*, a combination of contact and verbal exploration is needed before any improvement is seen over the control group. For *b*, each factor taken alone decreases distress; combined, they are somewhat better but not so good as would be expected if the two factors added together; for *c* both factors appear to increase distress, though when combined, they are about as effective in reducing distress as the control.

For each case the overall statistical test must be combined with a careful examination of pattern and supplemented by tests between specific pairs of conditions. Correct prediction of the pattern *prior* to the experiment greatly facilitates testing between pairs, as one can use a standard *t* test. But if the pattern is not anticipated, one should use more conservative multiple comparison tests. To reach a given level of significance the differences between conditions must be larger for these tests than for *t* tests. This takes into account the fact that we are more likely to find a significant effect if we compute all possible comparisons; e.g., six comparisons can be made between the four groups, though only three of these six tests are independent [93].

SITUATIONAL CONFOUNDS

Patients in a sample nearly always show variation on a wide number of factors that could have an observable effect on their responses to the experimental treatment [38]. By measuring such factors before data collection, one can assign patients to treatment groups in such a way that the factor occurs equally often in all groups.

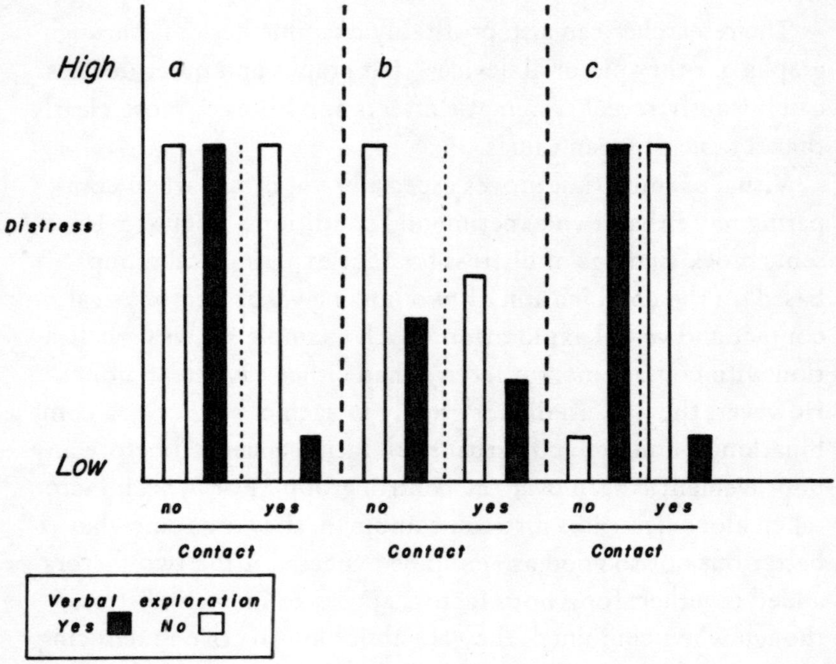

Fig. 5-1. Three hypothetical examples of levels of distress produced by interactions of contact and verbal exploration.

However, when these factors operate during the experiment (e.g., variables like length of anesthesia), one has no assurance that groups formed before surgery will be equivalent on these factors afterward. If we are lucky and these situational factors are equally distributed across treatments, the analysis proceeds directly; we can either ignore the factors, treating them as sources of error, or examine their contribution to the dependent variables by means of correlations or by using the situational factor as a variable in the data analysis. Of course, if treatments and situational factors are completely confounded (e.g., all patients receiving an experimental nursing treatment receive more anesthesia than controls), then one cannot draw a conclusion about the effects of the nursing treatments on postoperative recovery independent of the anesthesia. Where situational factors fall short of equal distribution across conditions, one can treat data with other techniques (see Winer [93]). Situational factors that could affect the data can often be identified from research reports relevant to the problem and from the clinical literature.

CHANGE SCORES

Change scores, the difference between an initial and subsequent level for a variable, are frequently used in behavioral research. In a study of nursing effects on anxiety during hospital admission, change scores are the difference between prenursing and post-nursing distress scores (see, for example, Mertz [71] and Anderson [1]). The score gives an estimate of the consequences of the nursing treatment. Every score consists of two components: a systematic component and a chance component, i.e., error or noise. A statistical test states the likelihood that chance rather than the systematic component produced the findings of difference.

There are many sources of error in experimental data. For example, a nurse-investigator may compare the intensity and number of behavioral signs of stress for each of two nursing conditions. She then asks if the difference between the two conditions is significantly greater than the error. When people are assigned to experimental treatment groups by random procedures, the variation within conditions is a good estimate of error (and is used as such in parametric statistical tests). This variation springs in part from a host of uncontrolled factors. These may include variations in the procedures used in the "same" nursing treatment; individual differences in susceptibility to the treatment; differences in the sources of their distress; and variations in the context in which the study is conducted. An important reason for using change scores is to allow us to control for some portion of this error by assessing the effects of a manipulation or a treatment *independent* of differences between individuals.

Unfortunately, some of the defects of change scores stem from their very advantage. For example, an investigator may use change scores to determine whether one nursing condition reduces stress more completely than another. One of her experimental nursing treatments produces a significantly large average change, but the other does not. She therefore concludes that the two conditions are not equivalent and assumes that the experimental condition successfully reduces stress. But suppose the experimenter, working as she is with difference scores, fails to examine the initial or final scores themselves, and let us assume that the group showing the larger change had much higher initial scores than the group showing the smaller change. Given large differences in initial level, the change scores may simply reflect the fact that high initial scores are more changeable than low initial scores. There are two bases for such an expectation. First, extreme scores, whether extremely high or extremely low, are susceptible to statistical regression on repeated measurement; i.e., our best prediction of a second score is closer to the mean of the distribution. Second, no human process can sustain itself at extremely high levels of activity over long periods of time. Therefore a very high distress will probably move downward, regardless of nursing procedure. An additional concern in comparing change scores when the initial scores are unequal is that the comparison requires an interval scale in order to say that the larger of the changes is actually bigger. Unfortunately, we can seldom prove that the units are equal at all places along our scales.

It is important, then, for the investigator to examine the initial level of scores in her experimental groups, regardless of the type of response she measures. Differences in initial levels may effect change independently of, or in interaction with, actual experimental effects, in levels of opinions, feelings, attitudes [23] and in various physiological measures such as heart rate and palmar conductance [45, 48, 49, 62].

Another example illustrates the absurd conclusions that can be drawn when experimenters fail to take account of initial levels of scores. Suppose we designed a study to assess the relative merits of two procedures for educating nurses on how to care for maternity patients and discovered that for one method, individuals learn more quickly and learn more than in the other. Subtracting measures of the final level of retention two weeks later from immediate postlearning measures to get retention scores, we would probably find that individuals who have learned quickly learn more and forget more than those who learned little. Does this mean that amount retained is inversely related to rate of learning? Perhaps, but we must remember that those nurses who learned much had more to forget. In fact, one who learned absolutely nothing would show no forgetting on the second test! In cases such as this, investigators may try to develop special ratio scores – change relative to change possible – but these, too, have problems.

Dealing with change scores is a difficult business, and one must proceed with caution. The following example illustrates another pitfall. Suppose we wish to compare the effects of two nursing treatments for reduction of postsurgical distress and discover that by chance, or malevolent fate, average initial distress level is lower in the experimental nursing group (*E*) than in the comparison control (*C*). We may decide to eliminate the initial difference by matching our groups after we have collected the data. To do this we would select patients with high initial scores from group *E* and patients with low initial scores from *C*. Unfortunately, if we then compared our matched groups, the comparison could be invalid, as we have confounded our comparison with regression effects [15]. Since we chose high scores from *E* and low scores from *C*, we can predict that had we taken a second measure without applying any treatment whatsoever, the two groups would be likely to differ as we would expect the second set of *E* scores to be lower and the second set of *C* scores to be higher; the best prediction for any second measure is that it will be closer to the true population mean than the first. The correct strategy would have been first to match subjects on initial distress and then to randomly assign the members of the pair to the two nursing treatments. Matching pairs of subjects on some measure is a legitimate way to reduce error, but the subjects must first be matched and then placed in opposite groups by a random assignment procedure.

"CEILING" AND "FLOOR" EFFECTS

Other mechanical and statistical artifacts are important for change scores and single measures as well. Problems comparing change scores can arise, due to "floor" or "ceiling" effects. Thus when initial scores are already at or near the bottom of a scale, it is difficult for them to move downward. The measuring instrument cannot detect changes in both directions equally well. To a degree the investigator can deal with such problems if she anticipates them. If she realized she is studying stress reduction in situations where initial stress is relatively mild, she should use measuring instruments with high sensitivity in the low stress range. This caution holds even if single scores are taken after the treatments and change scores are not computed. When one uses physiological measures for distress, one must attend carefully to departures from optimal or homeostatic level; the size and direction of such departures affects the size and direction of change to environmental alterations. For example, hypertensive patients will be more likely to show large decreases in blood pressure and hypotensive or normotensive patients, little or no decreases, or pehaps even increases as they return to resting level. If a nursing treatment should move patients to a stable homeostatic level, an investigator might not detect the treatment's effect using simple directional change scores in so complex a sample.

NONEQUIVALENCE OF THE METRIC

Most of the problems we have discussed involve the fundamental issue of whether units are of equal size at different points on the metric. The various problems of the equivalence of units stem from the fact that nearly all of the analysis procedures and theoretical points assume the possibility of measurement by interval scales. If this assumption is false, the seriousness of the error will depend on the conclusion drawn from the specific findings. For example, if she compares only two groups of subjects, the investigator needs to say little more than whether or not the two groups differ; the unit of difference is of little significance.

More complex problems arise with complex designs; e.g., in studies comparing two types of nursing care for two different medical procedures. Designs of this sort are very efficient, allowing one to compare the effects of several procedures on different types of cases all with just one set of data. But these designs usually require the investigator to evaluate complex interactions; i.e., she not only compares the two types of nursing procedures with one another and the two types of medical procedures with one another, but also looks to see if the differences between the two types of nursing are more pronounced for one medical procedure than for the other. This test involves a comparison of two differences and is appropriate only when the two differences are based on the same scale unit. If the investigator measures the same response, e.g., heart rate or facial changes, she can all too easily assume she is using the same unit, but this may not be so. Let us take a hypothetical example:

Suppose two types of medical procedures, surgery and radiation therapy, show different initial response levels, surgery producing a higher level of posttreatment discomfort than a focused radiation treatment. This could produce a larger difference between the nursing care procedures after surgery (a difference, say, of 18 beats per minute versus 8) and could suggest greater value in using the superior nursing treatment in surgical cases. If, however, the true scale unit is very large at high levels of distress (a change of 18 heart beats per minute at 140 beats could actually be a smaller distress change than 8 beats per minute at 80), then the difference between the nursing treatments is actually larger for patients receiving the radiation treatment. Adopting the preferred treatment would actually provide a significantly more noticeable change for the radiation cases.

Another problem caused by differences in scale unit size arises when we form a scale by combining scores from two different measures. Investigators often form such scales from sets of attitude items. In adding the items, the investigator may assume that the scale units are equal for each item simply because they all use seven-point scales, but this assumption is unwarranted. For one item, subjects or judges may cluster about only three scale steps, while for another they may spread over the full range of the scale. If she simply adds the two responses, the one with the greater spread has relatively greater weight in the sum. This can be more easily seen when we consider the extreme case where every patient gets the same score for one of two questions; when the two scores are summed, the differences between patients will be determined entirely by the single item where they differ.

A variety of techniques help us handle unequal scale units. We can transform raw scores into standard score units so that every person's score for each measure is expressed in terms of deviations in standardized steps from the group mean, and the variation about the mean is equal (one unit) for all measures. Other methods determine whether the scale unit is of equal size throughout the metric and are discussed in detail in volumes on scale scaling [30, 87]. The problem of initial values, an important one in our example of computing change scores for heart rate, is considered in a variety of ways in psychophysiology [45, 48, 49] and in attitude measurement [80]. Usually, one computes change as some proportion of the initial level or of the amount of potential change on the available scale. Unfortunately, none of the solutions is perfect, and the investigator should turn to these sources and examine their solutions with some care if she suspects she faces problems of a shifting metric.

Times Series Designs

We have discussed the value of examining time trends for individual subjects separately, and the various problems involved in the use of change scores. Our discussion so far has assumed that comparisons could be made between time series data for two or more groups. But there are special circumstances under which the standard experimental design is difficult if not impossible to run. Perhaps a promising, untested experimental treatment cannot be withheld from patients because all prior evidence shows that the control or substitute treatments are inadequate and perhaps fatal. Or perhaps, wishing to evaluate a new community-based mental health program or a state-wide auto safety campaign, the investigator can find no other community or state that matches the experimental group or cannot afford the costs of collecting such data. Or, having cleared even these hurdles, she can make no clearly valid conclusions through traditional procedures because one cannot compare a single experimental community to a single control community; there is no sample of communities to permit the calculation of experimental error. What can be done?

Fortunately, the investigator can employ other procedures to help her determine whether or not the experimental treatment has measurably affected her group. Basically, she needs historical or statistical records from which she can generate time series data and compare the course of events immediately subsequent to the introduction of the treatment with events prior to it. Figure 5-2, taken from Campbell and Stanley [15], illustrates eight possible shapes of the time series data obtained from eight sequential observations; these could be eight years of accident statistics, eight months or eight weeks of death rates from a disease.

In each instance (curves *A* through *H*) the experimental treatment is applied (at *X*) between the fourth and fifth observation. In all eight of the curves a rise follows the application of the treatment, but only *A* and *B* strongly indicate that the treatment is responsible for the increment. Curves *A* and *B* rise sharply soon

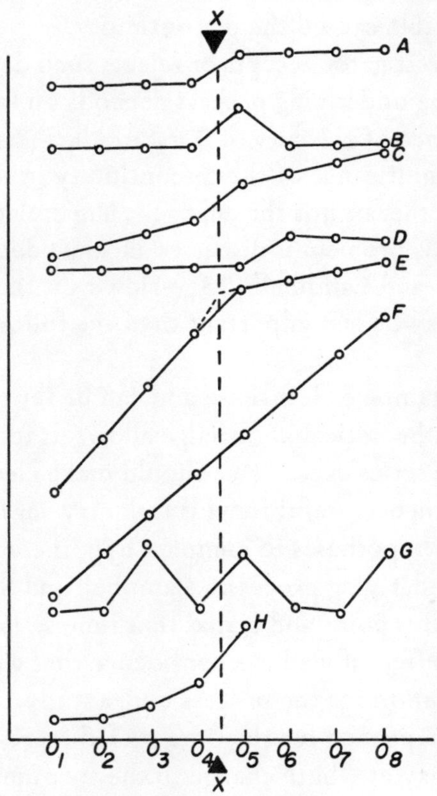

Fig. 5-2. Some possible outcome patterns from the introduction of an experimental variable at point *X* into a time series of measurements – observations 1 to 8 (0_1 to 0_8). Except for example *D*, the 0_4 to 0_5 gain is the same for all the time series, while the legitimacy of inferring an effect varies widely, being strongest in examples *A* and *B* and totally unjustified in examples *F, G,* and *H*. (Adapted from Campbell and Stanley [15].)

after the application of the treatment, but *A* then flattens out while *B* declines. Curve *F*, which rises throughout, or *H*, which begins to rise prior to the application of treatment, does not suggest that the treatment is responsible for the change in the measures. The key features of curves *A* and *B* are (1) the rise occurs immediately after and contiguous with the application of the treatment, and (2) no other signs of change occur at other points on the curve. Curve *C* also seems to meet our test, as there is a break in the trajectory or slope of the curve contiguous with the application of the treatment. Here, however, the continuous rise suggests the operation of some other variable, and there is the risk that this variable caused the discontinuity.

Whether an investigator accepts or rejects such data as evidence for a change in the underlying process depends on factors other than the appearance of the curves. First of all, a statistical test must assess the significance of the discontinuity in slope; this would tell us whether or not the change is large relative to chance expectations. This problem is discussed in some detail by Campbell and Stanley [15] and Campbell [13]. However, these statistical considerations may be less important than the following theoretical ones.

Time series data make clear sense and can be rationally interpreted when our theoretical knowledge allows us to predict the shape of the time series curve. (We should make clear, however, that the level of theory useful for this task may vary widely from simple, empirical hypotheses to complex hypotheses derived from a model of the underlying process.) Campbell and Stanley [15] also emphasized this point and stated that time series data indicate a treatment effect if we have confidence that we have achieved *experimental isolation* for the process under study. In short, if nothing else has happened for the time period represented by the data points, we may attribute change to the treatment.

It is obviously more difficult to achieve experimental isolation for some processes and problems than for others, e.g., for the state-wide safety campaign [13] in comparison with a new nursing treatment. Isolation is a function of many factors! In the physics laboratory it can be achieved by instruments. In a field setting, such control is only achievable by statistical examination of possible confounds and fairly precise specification of the predicted treatment effect. To rule out confounds, one examines all other factors that might influence the data. For example, for the safety campaign one must ask were there more or fewer cars on the road each year? Were there shifts in the age, social class, and training of drivers? Interpretation is simplified in the absence of such factors of change. But even if such variables are present, one can see if their onset immediately precedes changes in the time series; if not, one can probably rule them out as significant to the change process.

A model of the process can also strengthen inference. For example, curve *A* in Figure 5-2, an upswing followed by a plateau, is reasonable if the treatment, such as a new drug or new care procedure, remains in effect or is expected to have lasting effects (such as an intensive or continuing educational program). Curve *B*, a rise and fall, is more reasonable for many processes that offer temporary incentives and pressures for change, but do not create mechanisms for lasting effects; e.g., as a mass media campaign for safety or a group drive to curb smoking.

Curve *H* is especially interesting as it suggests that the change process predates the treatment. A change of this sort may appear when the treatment is psychological or behavioral, and the experimenters or practitioners being trained in the procedure know that it will be applied at time *X*. Thus, in studies of nursing care, when the behavior of the nurse is a source of information or reinforcement for the patient, such an effect suggests that the treatment itself may be irrelevant and that the important factors may be the demeanor and expressive behavior of the practitioner. One must have a control group to help interpret curve *H*, as by itself it merely suggests that the changes are independent of the treatment. Such an effect can be seen in a study by Leventhal and Fischer [57], in which the behavior of the experimenters apparently changed in *anticipation* of the treatments and altered subject performance.

Clearly, time series data offer many ways of testing manipulations in the absence of control comparisons. And clearly, the precision of interpretation depends on the shape of the curve and its fit to theoretical expectations. Thus the interpretation of time series data demonstrates once again that selection and interpretation of measures are intimately tied to our theoretical conception of the process under study. Most processes have a broad range of effects and a fairly broad range of measures; a public safety campaign, the introduction of brake inspection stations, and so on, will probably influence accident records, but one can look at accident records in several ways, and some ways may be better for detecting our treatment effects. Unfortunately, practitioners and administrators concerned with impressive statistics, such as reduction of accidental deaths, may select dependent measures inappropriate for detecting the consequences of their programs. For example, there may be too few accidents due to brake failures for brake inspection to reduce death statistics. The best criterion of program success may be the number of faulty brakes encountered over successive weeks of the program.

A similar issue exists in introducing a new nursing or informational program into the hospital. Suppose we want to prepare patients for surgery and apply our treatment uniformly to all patients. Here, it would probably be unwise to use a dependent measure such as postoperative complications, since complications may be few and only distantly related to postoperative emotional disturbance and the ease with which the patient can manage himself following surgery. We might better record the amounts of pain medication used, as this measure comes closer to the process under study. In short, the investigator must consider her measures in terms of proximity to the process she is trying to influence and the degree to which the indicator is likely to be affected by other variables operating in the setting. Possibly, each of her measures responds to a variety of influences; the investigator should then select a measure that is maximally responsive to the manipulated variables and minimally responsive to possible confounding factors. In short, she should try to select a measure that is likely to yield curves like *A* or *B* in Figure 5-2 and avoid indicators she knows are likely to show steady rises or falls or other abrupt shifts due to changes in variables other than those under study.

Comments on Statistics

The investigator must weigh the appropriateness of the statistical analysis for the measures she uses. The warning is frequently sounded that only such techniques as the chi-square or comparisons between proportions should be applied to frequency (category) data. On the other hand, *t* tests and analysis of variance are said to be inapplicable to anything less than interval data. Rather than warn the investigator to use a less efficient technique, we prefer to emphasize using the most powerful statistic possible. A test of low power can fail to identify a difference when one exists and can lead to the conclusion that the treatment had no effect when in fact it did. Data often adequately meet the assumptions of more powerful statistical tests, and the investigator should be loathe to throw away information contained in her data. Moreover, one need not meet all of the assumptions of the interval scale to use parametric tests [33]. We can use *t* tests or analysis of variance without equal-size scale units, as long as we do not discuss differences between groups as if the magnitude of the differences could be treated as known.

The issue of power, or ability to detect differences caused by treatments, relates to more factors than the sensitivity of the statistical measure used. When experimental treatments are very strong, they are obviously more likely to produce large and therefore significant differences when compared with control groups. But a comparison between a relatively weak treatment and a control may yield a highly significant difference if the sample is large enough. One hears much about the merits of small versus large samples, both pro and con. The great merit of large samples, at least for nursing research, is that the investigator can subdivide her subjects within treatment conditions and examine the effects of other factors such as social class, type of medication, and physician in charge. Such situational and background factors are not of direct interest, but the variability they introduce into the data may be very great, and their impact can be assessed statistically only if there is a reasonable number of cases. The hope that random assignment equalizes samples on all such factors is too often only a hope.

The merit of small samples, paradoxically, is that one can almost always find a statistically reliable effect if the sample is large enough [7, 61]. The investigator must distinguish between the statistical significance of an effect (whether it may be due to chance) and the meaningfulness of the effect, i.e., whether or not it is big enough to make a difference. A good theory can predict whether an effect should be small or large; indeed, when quantification has proceeded to an advanced stage so that both treatments and responses are scaled, theory should predict the size of the difference expected. The experimenter should have some idea of the likely size of his effects and should choose a sample size and a probability level (a level of significance at which he will reject the null hypothesis) appropriate for the magnitude of the expected effect.

Improvement in predictive power is not mere window dressing; indeed, for nursing research, in which results have practical implications, the relative size of the effects produced by different treatments compared with their cost and effort needs to be considered in a decision framework to optimize patient care. It helps to know that *A* is better than *B* and that *C* is better than *D*. But if we wish to choose a combination of three or four treatments from among a large number of possibilities, it helps to know how much better, how much cost and time, and whether the same or greater benefit could be derived from dropping one costly treatment and adding two less expensive ones.

A number of statistical devices help answer questions about the meaningfulness of findings as distinct from their statistical significance. These descriptive indices resemble correlation coefficients. A correlation coefficient, such as the Pearson product moment r, varies from +1.0 through 0 to −1.0, and describes the degree of association between two factors. Thus the correlation tells how much of the variability in one measure can be accounted for by variability in the other when the scores are expressed in standard score units. Correlation-like indices can be computed in the analysis of variance [93] and tell how much of the variability in the data derives from systematic effects of the treatments. If such an index shows that 50 percent of the variation in a set of distress scores is associated with the differences between two nursing treatments, the investigator knows that the treatments account for a very substantial portion of the between-person variability.

Since these indices express the proportion of variance accounted for, the same size proportion can be found under quite different circumstances. For example, a comparison between experimental and control nursing could account for 50 percent of the variance when the two groups differ only moderately, and there is relatively little variability within the groups. Such a case might occur when distress is not very high to begin with. The same ratio could also occur in a comparison in which the control group showed much higher distress than the experimental group and the variability within the groups was high, a likely case when distress is very great. Although in both of the examples the experimental treatment reduces the same amount of distress relative to the variability in distress present in the study sample, the high distress cases in the control group and exceptionally low distress in the experimental condition make for a dramatic contrast. Thus practitioners who tend to focus on the individual case rather than the overall effects might be more impressed by the latter study, though both offer impressive evidence in favor of the experimental nursing care.

One should note two important cautions in the use of coefficients of association. First, a correlation measures *association*, not *causation*. Correlated factors may be causally related (i.e., changing one factor produces changes in the other), but mere statistical association does not prove causation. Second, if one uses several dependent measures in an experimental study, one should probably examine their independence by computing correlations between them. Three types of correlations can be calculated: (1) correlations between measures across all subjects, an overall *r*; (2) correlations between measures where the scores are the *means for the conditions* in the experiment (not useful if there are only two conditions, as the correlation can only take one of three values, namely, +1.0, 0.0, or −1.0); and (3) correlations between measures computed separately for the subjects within each of the experimental conditions. The first type of correlation, across all subjects, is often used to estimate the association between measures in experiments. But it is a misleading estimate when reported to supplement the analysis of the difference between treatment means; this is so because this correlation includes the treatment effects. For example, if both dependent measures are high in some conditions and low in others, a significant *r* will be found for all subjects even though within any condition there is no association between the factors.

A PRIORI AND POST HOC TESTS

Many investigators take the position that data should be examined only for predictions stated in advance. We would not limit statistical treatment in this way. Rather, we suggest the researcher look at her data for unexpected occurrences or relationships and test these with statistics that take into account that the prediction was not made beforehand (e.g., see Hays [33], pp. 488–490). She should then predict other relationships that would be found in the data if the new findings are valid (for example, the predictions may suggest rearranging the categories of the data, or finding correlations of one set of items with another, using data on the effectiveness of the experimental manipulations). These new predictions are then tested with appropriate statistical procedures.

Many experimenters believe that an ex post facto finding should not be published until verified by further research. While this is technically correct, it may be unrealistic and does not fully use available data. When the researcher is conservative in approach, i.e., uses post hoc tests and makes other predictions regarding the data at hand that are borne out in further analyses, she has stronger support for her findings and can provide a compelling reason for others to follow through with further research. Field experiments consume time and money, and the investigator must take full advantage of her data set. The cost and time of these studies, however, also demand careful analysis of both theoretical assumptions and situations, pretesting of procedures and measures, and as precise a statement of predictions as possible. Indeed, one should often break a large study into a series of smaller investigations, so that later designs and methods can benefit from earlier ones.

RELIABILITY

One contributor to error variance is the nonrepeatability or unreliability of the measuring instruments. Most instruments for measuring behavior are imperfect; i.e., their readings will vary from trial to trial even though the underlying or true score remains constant. A variety of methods help assess the reliability of a measuring device and can be used to identify techniques having excessive error variance. If unreliability is very large relative to the magnitude of the events measured, one should usually discard the instrument. Cronbach [16] discusses these questions of reliability in detail.

Two main techniques exist for computing reliability, the so-called split-half (or odd-even, another version of the same approach) method and the test-retest method. In deciding which to use, the investigator must consider a variety of theoretical questions about the underlying behavioral process. For example, if she wishes to assess a personality trait, a competency factor (e.g., intelligence), or any factor assumed to be a relatively unvarying attribute of a human being, then she should assess the variable at points relatively removed in time (test-retest methods). If she is concerned with fluctuating processes, such as distress, emotional state, or moods, it seems less reasonable to use the test-retest technique, as this measure involves the reliability of the subject's interpretation of the setting as much as the reliability of the measures. The concept guides our choice of reliability assessment, and there is no simple rule for choosing the best reliability technique for a given process. Blind adherence to one or another technique can result in artifically higher or lower estimates of consistency, depending on which other factors are permitted to vary.

AGREEMENT AMONG JUDGES

When judges score behavior either directly in the setting or from a record such as a television picture, the problem of reliability becomes one of inter-judge agreement. Judges can agree for a variety of reasons, not all of which are meaningful. One must consider the basis of agreement when computing reliability. For example, judges may agree because they accurately judge all of the responses being coded (an ideal case), or because they agree on some particular patient(s). As an example, let us assume that the judges are rating 10 indicators of distress and that two of these appear much more frequently than the others. Extremely high agreement among the judges could reflect agreement on only those responses. One or all of the less frequent indicators may have low inter-judge agreement (which is impossible to determine if they are very infrequent). If the instrument is then used in a new situation where the low-frequency indicators appear regularly, the effectiveness of the system will at best be questionable.

Or, let us suppose that a small number of patients produced the major proportion of the distress responses. High reliability could reflect agreement in scoring these patients, while agreement may be very low for those patients who produced few indicators of distress. If the low reliability for the remaining patients is not merely a reflection of an extremely small number of judgments, it may mean that only some types of people can be judged with consistency.

In some cases, inter-judge agreement is highest for responses that occur with high and nearly equal frequency in all patients; i.e., the very responses that do not discriminate between patients with different degrees of distress. On the other hand, the few responses that actually discriminate between nursing conditions may show low inter-rater agreement. Similarly, patients for whom there is high agreement may be patients who show little or no reaction to the experimental procedures.

In both cases, then, the conclusions to be drawn about experimental nursing techniques depend on the least reliable responses. Under such conditions one can expect experimental results to show low replicability, and the investigator may conclude that particular nursing procedures are ineffective simply because her measuring instrument lacked reliability for these key indicators. In summary, reliability must be computed for that category of response that is critical for assessing the impact of experimental nursing procedures.

RESEARCH STRATEGY

It is not enough to think about and resolve problems at each of the conceptual, observational, and analytical steps that have been discussed. The researcher also must be aware of the relatedness between them. The planning and execution of research does not go in a straight line from concept through observation to analysis, but moves back and forth through all of them.

This may seem complicated, and it is, especially in a relatively new field of research. In a highly advanced scientific discipline, concepts are well defined and carry with them an accepted framework of measurement along with a technology for data management. Newer disciplines show less agreement between investigators on the definition of appropriate concepts. The operations used are many and changing; data treatment varies and tends to be less precise; and the statistical techniques used are less powerful. The field of behavioral research exhibits much imprecision in definition and procedures. While this is not surprising, it can be discouraging, so that a researcher is tempted to do "clean" research and to work only on those questions that permit the most rigorous methods.

It is easy for an investigator to make the above choice if she views the scientific enterprise as analogous to the assembly of a picture puzzle in which her job is to assemble the pieces and see the picture on the box. But this view may be oversimplified and erroneous. Scientific work does involve putting together many pieces, but the analogy must be sharply modified because there is no clear picture on the box to tell us what the final product will be. Indeed, the most interesting part of the game is when the picture changes while one is building the puzzle. However, the presence of what Kuhn [43] has called scientific revolutions, or sharp changes in our view of the picture, sets very stringent methodological and theoretical requirements for the investigator. In order to know whether the picture (theory) is changing or her method is failing, she must state her theories as precisely as she can and use the most rigorous methods possible. Under such conditions she can move toward constructing a model that reasonably approximates reality.

It is important, however, to keep in mind that the aim of nursing research is to use theory and method to solve practice problems. To do this one must be prepared to grapple with both refined and ambiguous concepts, with techniques of measurement both neat and "messy," and with methods of data analysis both rigorous and "weak." We must use the best methods appropriate to our problems, but we cannot choose our problems solely because of available methodology. The practical problems posed by distress due to illness and treatment and the broad range of phenomena covered by nursing action define a host of socially and theoretically significant problems that demand investigation. These problems remain our basic challenge even if we lack the concepts and methods to easily define and investigate the phenomena underlying them. Indeed, the nurse-researcher may be fortunate in having a practice pressure that helps define and limit her activities as the pressure of practice can be protection against sterile research; i.e., research that is content to use precise methods to study meaningless concepts.

ACKNOWLEDGMENTS

The authors are especially indebted to Florence Wald and Robert Leonard for introducing them to the area of nursing research and stimulating them to prepare this material. Special thanks are also extended to Jean Johnson, who made several valuable comments and additions, and to Barbara Ellingson-Waugh for the editorial reworking of the final draft. The preparation of this material was supported by the United States Public Health Service, grant NU 00183-02.

NOTES

1. A researcher sometimes assumes a common concept and combines two or more measures without first checking to see how they are correlated. With a well-grounded body of theory and evidence, this may be justifiable; but lacking these, the researcher must examine for herself the relationship of her measures before combining scores in any way.

2. One might also argue that the internal validity of the experiment was reduced. Thus, if the observer increased the intensity of the pleasant and unpleasant states [79], and if the treatment's effect depended on this intensification, the observer is then a necessary condition for the success of the treatments. A conclusion interpreting the effect solely in terms of the treatment and illness stressors would be in error. On the other hand, the observer might simply intensify the effect in the particular indicators recorded, especially if they are expensive, and have no impact on internal or subjective state. The theoretical interpretation of this latter case is complex.

REFERENCES

1. Anderson, B. A study of the effect of the nurse's activity on the blood pressure readings, pulse rates, and comfort of patients admitted to a state mental hospital. Unpublished Master's report, Yale University School of Nursing, 1963.
2. Anderson, B., Mertz, H., and Leonard, R. C. Two experimental tests of a patient-centered admission process. *Nursing Research* 14:151–157, 1965.
3. Atkinson, J. W. *Motives in Fantasy, Action and Society.* Princeton: Van Nostrand, 1958.
4. Atkinson, J. W. *An Introduction to Motivation.* New York: Van Nostrand, 1964, pp. 240–267.
5. Atkinson, J. W., and Litwin, G. H. Achievement motive and test anxiety conceived as motive to approach success and motive to avoid failure. *Journal of Abnormal and Social Psychology* 60:52–63, 1960.
6. Ax, A. F. The physiological differentiation between fear and anger in humans. *Psychosomatic Medicine* 15:433–442, 1953.
7. Bakan, D. The test of significance in psychological research. *Psychological Bulletin* 66:423–437, 1966.
8. Barron, M. A. The effects varied nursing approaches have on patients' complaints of pain: a clinical experiment. Unpublished Master's report, Yale University School of Nursing, 1964.
9. Bartley, S. H. *Principles of Perception.* New York: Harper & Row, 1958.
10. Beecher, H. K. Pain in men wounded in battle. *Annals of Surgery* 123:96–105, 1946.
11. Beecher, H. K. *Measurement of Subjective Responses.* New York: Oxford University Press, 1959.
12. Brown, Roger. *Social Psychology.* New York: Free Press, 1965.
13. Campbell, D. T. Reforms as experiments. *American Psychologist* 24:409–429, 1969.
14. Campbell, D. T., and Fiske, D. W. Convergent and discriminant validation by the multitrait-multimethod matrix. *Psychological Bulletin* 56:81–105, 1959.
15. Campbell, D. T., and Stanley, J. C. *Experimental and Quasi-experimental Designs for Research on Teaching.* Chicago: Rand McNally, 1963.
16. Cronbach, L. J. *Essentials of Psychological Testing.* New York: Harper & Row, 1960.
17. Cronbach, L. J., and Meehl, P. E. Construct validity in psychological tests. *Psychological Bulletin* 52:281–302, 1955.
18. Dember, W. *The Psychology of Perception.* New York: Holt, Rinehart and Winston, 1960.
19. Edwards, A. *The Social Desirability Variable in Personality Assessment and Research.* New York: Dryden, 1957.
20. Edwards, A. *Experimental Design in Psychological Research.* New York: Holt, Rinehart and Winston, 1962.
21. Elder, R. G. A study of patients; verbal communications to the nurse.

Unpublished Master's report, Yale University School of Nursing, 1960.
22. Elms, R. R. The effects of varied nursing approaches during elective admission to a surgical unit. Unpublished Master's report, Yale University School of Nursing, 1963.
23. Festinger, L., and Katz, D. *Research Methods in the Behavioral Sciences.* New York: Dryden, 1953.
24. Frijda, N. H. Recognition of Emotion. In L. Berkowitz (Ed.), *Advances in Experimental Social Psychology* 4:343–352, 1969.
25. Galanter, E. Contemporary Psychophysics. In R. Brown et al. (Eds.), *New Directions in Psychology*, vol. I. New York: Holt, Rinehart and Winston, 1962, pp. 87–156.
26. Garner, W. R. Rating scales, discriminability, and information transmission. *Psychological Review* 67:343–352, 1960.
27. Garner, W. R., Hake, H. H., and Erickson, C. W. Operationism and the concept of perception. *Psychological Review* 63:149–159, 1956.
28. Grace, W. J., and Graham, D. T. Relationship of specific attitudes and emotions to certain bodily diseases. *Psychosomatic Medicine* 14:243–251, 1952.
29. Graham, D. T., Stern, J. A., and Winokur, G. Experimental investigation of the specificity of attitude hypothesis in psychosomatic disease. *Psychosomatic Medicine* 20:446–457, 1958.
30. Guilford, J. P. *Psychometric Methods.* New York: McGraw-Hill, 1954.
31. Hanawalt, N. G. The role of the upper and lower parts of the face as the basis for judging facial expressions, II. In posed expressions and "candid camera" pictures. *Journal of General Psychology* 31:23–36, 1944.
32. Hardy, J. D., and Javert, C. T. Studies on pain: measurements of pain intensity in childbirth. *Journal of Clinical Investigation* 28:153–162, 1949.
33. Hays, W. L. *Statistics for Psychologists.* New York: Holt, Rinehart and Winston, 1963.
34. Heckhausen, H. Achievement Motive Research: Current Problems and Some Contributions Towards a General Theory of Motivation. In W. V. Arnold (Ed.), *Nebraska Symposium on Motivation.* Lincoln: University of Nebraska Press, 1968, pp. 103–174.
35. Heyns, R. W., and Zander, A. F. Observation of Group Behavior. In L. Festinger, and D. Katz, (Eds.), *Research Methods in the Behavioral Sciences.* New York: Dryden, 1953, pp. 381–417.
36. Holsti, O. R., Loomba, J. K., and North, R. C. Content Analysis. In G. Lindzey and E. Aronson (Eds.), *The Handbook of Social Psychology* (2nd ed.), vol. 2. Reading, Mass.: Addison-Wesley, 1968.
37. Janis, I. L., and Leventhal, H. Human Reaction to Stress. In E. Borgatta and W. Lambert (Eds.), *Handbook of Personality Theory and Research.* Chicago: Rand McNally, 1968.
38. Johnson, B. A., Johnson, J. E., and Dumas, R. G. Research in nursing practice: The problem of uncontrolled situational variables. *Nursing Research* 19:337–342, 1970.
39. Johnson, J. E., and Leventhal, H. The effects of accurate expectations

and behavioral instructions on reactions during a noxious medical examination. *Journal of Personality and Social Psychology* 29:710–718, 1974.
40. Johnson, J., Leventhal, H., and Dabbs, J. M. Contribution of emotional and instrumental response processes in adaptation to surgery. *Journal of Personal and Social Psychology* 20:55–64, 1971.
41. Kaplan, A. *The Conduct of Inquiry.* San Francisco: Chandler, 1964.
42. Kornzweig, N. D. Behavior change as a function of fear arousal and personality. Unpublished doctoral dissertation, Yale University, 1967.
43. Kuhn, T. S. *The Structure of Scientific Revolutions* (2nd ed.). Chicago: University of Chicago Press, 1970.
44. Kushner, K. P. A study of the mood fluctuations of college females. Unpublished bachelor of arts thesis, University of Wisconsin, 1971.
45. Lacey, J. I. The evaluation of autonomic responses: toward a general solution. *Annals of the New York Academy of Sciences* 67:125–163, 1956.
46. Lacey, J. I. Somatic Response Patterning and Stress: Some Revisions of Activation Theory. In M. Appley and R. Trumbull (Eds.), *Psychological Stress.* New York: Appleton-Century-Crofts, 1967.
47. Lacey, J. I., Batemen, D. E., and Van Lehn, R. Autonomic response specificity: An experimental study. *Psychosomatic Medicine* 15:8–21, 1953.
48. Lacey, J. I., and Lacey, B. The law of initial value in the longitudinal study of autonomic response stereotype. *American Journal of Psychology* 71:50–73, 1958.
49. Lacey, J. I., and Lacey, B. The law of initial value in the longitudinal study of autonomic constitution: reproducibility of autonomic responses and response patterns over a four-year interval. *Annals of the New York Academy of Sciences* 98:1257–1290, 1962.
50. Lang, P. J. Fear Reduction and Fear Behavior: Problems in Treating a Construct. In J. M. Shlien (Ed.), *Research in Psychotherapy*, vol. III. Washington, D.C.: American Psychological Association, 1968, pp. 90–103.
51. Lazarus, R., and Alfert, E. Short-circuiting of threat by altering cognitive appraisal. *Journal of Abnormal and Social Psychology:* 69:195–205, 1966.
52. Leventhal, H. Fear – for your health. *Psychology Today* 1:55–58, 1967.
53. Leventhal, H. Experimental Studies in Anti-Smoking Communications. In E. Borgatta and R. Evans (Eds.), *Smoking, Health and Behavior.* Chicago: Aldine, 1968.
54. Leventhal, H. Findings and Theory in the Study of Fear Communications. In L. Berkowitz (Ed.), *Advances in Experimental Social Psychology.* New York: Academic, 1970, pp. 119–186.
55. Leventhal, H. Fear appeals and persuasion: The differentiation of a motivational construct. *American Journal of Public Health* 61:1208–1224, 1971.
56. Leventhal, H., Ellsberry, C., and Kedar, H. Measurement of emotion and its alteration by nursing. Mimeographed. Madison: University of Wisconsin. Progress report on grant NU-00302, 1969.

57. Leventhal, H., and Fischer, K. What reinforces in a social reinforcement situation – words or expression? *Journal of Personality and Social Psychology* 14:83–94, 1970.
58. Leventhal, H., and Niles, P. Persistence of influence for varying durations of exposure to threat stimuli. *Psychological Reports* 16:223–233, 1965.
59. Leventhal, H., and Sharp, E. Facial Expression and Distress. In S. S. Tomkins and C. I. Izard (Eds.), *Affect, Cognition and Personality.* New York: Springer, 1965.
60. Leventhal, H., Watts, J. C., and Pagano, F. Effects of fear and instructions on how to cope with danger. *Journal of Personality and Social Psychology* 6:313–321, 1967.
61. Lykken, D. T. Statistical significance in psychological research. *Psychological Bulletin* 70:151–159, 1968.
62. Lykken, T., Rose, R., Luther, B., and Malley, V. Correcting psychophysiological measures for individual differences in range. *Psychological Bulletin* 66:481–484, 1966.
63. Maccoby, E., and Maccoby, N. The Interview: A Tool of Social Science. In G. Lindzey (Ed.), *Handbook of Social Psychology,* vol. 1. Reading, Mass.: Addison-Wesley, 1954, pp. 449–487.
64. Malstrom, E. J., Opton, E. M., Jr., and Lazarus, R. S. Heart rate measurement and the correlation of indices of arousal. *Psychosomatic Medicine* 27:546–555, 1965.
65. Mandler, G. Stimulus variables and subject variables: A caution. *Psychological Review* 66:145–149, 1959.
66. McClelland, D. C., Atkinson, J. W., Clark, R. A., and Lowell, E. L. *The Achievement Motive.* New York: Appleton-Century-Crofts, 1953.
67. McGuire, W. J. Some impending reorientations in social psychology: Some thoughts provoked by Kenneth Ring. *Journal of Experimental Social Psychology* 3:123–139, 1967.
68. McNemar, Q. (Ed.) *Psychological Statistics.* New York: Wiley, 1962.
69. Melzack, R., and Casey, K. L. The Affective Dimension of Pain. In M. B. Arnold (Ed.), *Feelings and Emotions: The Loyola Symposium.* New York: Academic, 1970, pp. 55–68.
70. Melzack, R., and Wall, P. D. Pain mechanism: A new theory. *Science* 150:971–979, 1965.
71. Mertz, H. A study of the process of the nurse's activity as it affects the blood pressure readings and pulse rate of patients admitted to the emergency room. Unpublished Master's report, Yale University School of Nursing, 1961.
72. Miller, G. A. The magical number seven plus or minus two. *Psychological Review* 63:81–97, 1956.
73. Mischel, W. *Personality and Assessment.* New York: Wiley, 1968.
74. Orne, M. T. On the social psychology of the psychological experiment: With particular reference to demand characteristics and their implications. *American Psychology* 17:776–783, 1962.
75. Ring, K. Experimental social psychology: Some sober questions about some frivolous values. *Journal of Experimental Social Psychology* 3:113–123, 1967.

76. Rosen, T. J., and Leventhal, H. Two motives for smoking reduction, fear and danger. Mimeographed. Madison: University of Wisconsin, 1972.
77. Rosenthal, R. The effects of the experimenter on the results of psychological research. *Progress in Experimental Personality Research* 60:421–428, 1964.
78. Schacter, J. Pain, fear and anger in hypertensives and normotensives. *Psychosomatic Medicine* 19:17–29, 1957.
79. Schachter, S., and Singer, J. E. Cognitive, social, and psychological determinants of emotional state. *Psychological Review* 69:379–399, 1962.
80. Scott, W. A. Attitude Measurement. In G. Lindzey and E. Aronson (Eds.)., *The Handbook of Social Psychology* (2nd ed.), vol. 2. Reading, Mass.: Addison-Wesley, 1968.
81. Shapiro, D., and Crider, A. Psychophysiological Approaches in Social Psychology. In G. Lindzey, and E. Aronson (Eds.), *The Handbook of Social Psychology*, vol. 3. Reading, Mass.: Addison-Wesley, 1969, pp. 1–49.
82. Siegel, S. *Non-parametric Statistics for the Behavioral Sciences.* New York: McGraw-Hill, 1956.
83. Snedecor, G. W. *Statistical Methods.* Ames: Iowa State University Press, 1956.
84. Stevens, S. S. On the operation known as judgement. *American Scientist* 54:385–401, 1966.
85. Taylor, S., and Epstein, S. Measurement of autonomic arousal. *Psychosomatic Medicine* 29:514–525, 1967.
86. Tomkins, S. S. *Affect, Imagery, Consciousness,* vol. 1. *The Positive Affects.* New York: Springer Publishing Co., 1962.
87. Torgerson, W. S. *Theory and Methods of Scaling.* New York: Wiley, 1958.
88. Walker, H. M., and Lev, J. *Statistical Inference.* New York: Holt, Rinehart and Winston, 1953.
89. Walton, E. A. Hand and arm motor behavior in laboring patients. Unpublished Master's report, Yale University School of Nursing, 1967.
90. Webb, E. J., Campbell, D. T., Schwartz, R. D., and Sechrest, L. *Unobtrusive Method: Non-reactive Research in the Social Sciences.* Chicago: Rand McNally, 1966.
91. Weick, K. E. Systematic Observational Methods. In G. Lindzey and E. Aronson (Eds.), *The Handbook of Social Psychology* (2nd ed.), vol. 2. Reading, Mass.: Addison-Wesley, 1968.
92. Weiner, B. New Conceptions in the Study of Achievement Motivation. In B. S. Maher (Ed.), *Progress in Experimental Personality Research,* vol. 5. New York: Academic, 1970, pp. 67–109.
93. Winer, B. J. *Statistical Principles in Experimental Design.* New York: McGraw-Hill, 1962.
94. Woodworth, R., and Schlosberg, H. *Experimental Psychology.* New York: Holt, Rinehart and Winston, 1954.
95. Zajonc, R. B. Social facilitation. *Science* 149:269–274, 1965.

Research Related to Death and the Dying Patient

Jeanne Quint Benoliel

6

THIS chapter deals with some of the philosophical, methodological, and practical issues to be considered in designing and implementing research about sensitive and delicate matters in human affairs. In a sense, death is used as an example of a larger category of topics that pose difficulties for study because of their personal nature and the emotionally laden meanings associated with them. The discussion centers around the use of participant observation as a methodology for investigating the personal and social meanings of death and dying within a sociocultural context. The source from which much of the commentary derives is direct experience with the use of fieldwork in research designed to describe and understand how the phenomenon of death affected the lives of three different groups of people: women adjusting to mastectomy and the diagnosis of breast cancer; student nurses encountering death and dying as part of their introduction to becoming nurses; and young diabetics learning the psychosocial meanings of being diabetic.

DEATH AS A TOPIC FOR RESEARCH

In recent years, research into the psychological and sociological meanings of death has been initiated by investigators in several disciplines. The questions posed by each researcher were framed within the theoretical orientations of his special field of study. Thus the design and the methodology chosen in each case were guided by the types of data viewed as maximally useful for seeking answers to a particular set of questions. For example, to investigate attitudes toward death in the mentally ill, Feifel [16] developed a questionnaire that contained both direct and indirect questions about the meaning of death. To study the effects of death and dying on social relationships within the hospital, Glaser and Strauss [23, 25] collected data by using participant observation in several types of hospitals and then compared these findings for their similarities and differences. A similar approach was used by Sudnow [57] in his ethnography of death in a public hospital.

That nurses have an interest in death as a topic of clinical concern is clearly evident in the attention given to it in recent books and nursing journals. Active participation by nurses in both formal study and clinical investigation concerned with death and dying has been on the increase. Recognition that nurses feel inadequate to meet the psychosocial needs of dying patients was formally noted in an unpublished study by Bregg, Leddy, and MacKenzie [8] in 1953. Studying nurses' perceptions about the care of patients dying of cancer, Dickinson [13] reported that nurses feel insecure in meeting the religious needs of patients, in coping with patients who are completely helpless, and in dealing with families, especially those that are anxious, hostile, or constantly asking for information.

Using a sociological framework, Folta [17] found an ambivalent orientation toward death among hospital workers; it was viewed as peaceful and predictable in the abstract and with a high degree of anxiety when it became personalized. Both Smith [54] and Quint [43] reported that nursing students were taught about the physical and technical aspects of care of the dying but received little formalized direction for handling the psychosocial problems that appear in nursing practice. Waechter [59] found that children between the ages of six and ten, though not directly informed of the fact that they had a life-threatening illness, showed considerable preoccupation with death in fantasy, feelings of loneliness and isolation, and a sense of loss of control over the forces impinging upon them.

Interesting as are the findings that have been reported from these and other investigations, this chapter is not concerned with the substantive results of research about death and dying. Rather, its purpose is to describe the types of death-related problems that are amenable to study using participant observation as the preferred methodology and to consider some of the philosophical and pragmatic issues that come into play when this methodology is chosen.

THE PROBLEM TO BE STUDIED

As is true for many phenomena in which human beings have an interest, death is a subject that can be studied by either a deductive or an inductive approach. In the former case, some aspect of death is formulated as a theoretical construct within the context of a relatively well-defined theory. Certain characteristics or properties are selected as indicators of that construct in the empirical world. Instruments are selected or developed for collecting information that can then be used for judging whether or not the chosen properties can with confidence be accepted as "measurements" of the construct being investigated. Hooper and Spilka [30], for example, developed some Likert-type scales for collecting information about perspectives on future time and attitudes toward death from a sample of young people as part of a study to test the assumption that current beliefs and behaviors are directly related to perspectives about time and death.

In contrast to the approach just described, the investigator using an inductive approach examines death within a broad and rather loosely defined conceptual framework. Under the guidance of a set of orienting concepts, the researcher enters the field to collect empirical data about the phenomenon he has chosen to study. From the descriptive accounts of his observations, he formulates categories and propositions to use in speculating about the meanings and relationships existing among the theoretical constructs he has chosen for examination.

In inductive research, the methodology of participant observation is used for investigating death as part of a given social situation or complex social organization. The theoretical orientations underlying such studies are those formulated to describe and understand human behavior in social context. Thus, using the cultural anthropologist's perspective, Benedict [4] examined and interpreted death customs and practices (as well as other social customs) in primitive societies as reflections of fundamental beliefs and values held by these groups of people. A sociological interest in the relationships existing between social structure and social interaction guided Glaser and Strauss [23] in their analysis of the process of dying in hospitals. Symbolic interaction theory [7] that defines human beings as creatures who define and classify situations and people, including themselves, provided the theoretical framework for my own studies [5, 43] about the effects of death on the development of new identities.

Origins of a Problem

Although theory provides the framework for research, investigations do not appear out of thin air. Rather, they originate in subjective experiences that cause the investigator to ask questions about particular events. The mastectomy study, for example, came into being when the investigator (then an instructor of surgical nursing in a large medical center) began to wonder whether or not practitioners really knew very much about the "emotional needs" (a popular phrase at that time) of patients who had radical surgery of a disfiguring nature. Although interest was initially centered on the general phenomenon of surgical disfigurement, selection of mastectomy for the first project was undoubtedly influenced by the direct experience of having a breast biopsy.

Movement from the point of being interested in surgical disfigurement to the delineation of a researchable problem did not come about with ease, however. The process required a shift from the action-oriented perspective of a nurse looking at people as patients to the more reflective perspective of an investigator looking at people as human beings undergoing major psychosocial crises. Such a shift in orientation is both painful and difficult, but it is a necessary step in the development of a nurse-researcher. The goals, procedures, and intellectual operations of clinical practice are dissimilar and even sometimes in conflict with those of scientific observation and discovery of knowledge, as Gunter [27] has noted.

Typically, a formal problem develops through stages, beginning with an exploratory phase that one might consider as roughly equivalent to a pilot project. During periods of exploration, the investigator checks out some of his general hunches by collecting preliminary data that help him to clarify his thoughts about the problem and to sharpen the focus of his study. Prior to formalizing the study of adjustment following mastectomy, for instance, interviews were conducted with a number of women who had already undergone the experience of having a breast removed. These data were used to guide the subsequent statement of the problem, the overall approach chosen for the study, the sources to be sought for collecting data, and other procedural matters relative to research design.

Research Design

The restatement of the problem and the formulation of a research plan in keeping with the questions posed are facilitated when the investigator has access to knowledgeable, interested consultants who by their comments and questions force him to clarify the language and precision of his proposed investigation. In fact, the availability of well-selected consultants for the duration of the study is a critically important mechanism for helping the investigator to recognize bias and distortion in his observations and to make reasonable judgments about modifications and changes in procedure as unforeseen contingencies appear. Provision for appropriate and competent consultants is viewed as a necessary and vital component of research design for investigations that use participant observation as a methodology. Furthermore, several categories of consultation may be required if the study is concerned with knowledge derived from several disciplines.

Although preliminary data help to tighten the focus of the study, the research design for the type of investigation under discussion is still formulated with an open and flexible approach.

Broad rather than narrow guidelines and procedures are projected. A specific example, again taken from the mastectomy study [37], may illustrate the point more readily than additional commentary:

> The loss of an external part or mutilation such that there is deviation from the usual path for carrying out a normal physiologic function and usual everyday activities is a serious problem to many undergoing surgery. Radical mastectomy in women as one instance of the general phenomenon of surgical disfigurement has been selected as a problem which offers opportunity to investigate the process of adjustment which takes place when a woman is faced simultaneously with (1) loss of the breast, symbol of femininity and motherhood, and (2) invasion by a potentially destroying disease, cancer. Unlike limb amputations, this form of loss can be kept hidden except in circumstances involving a state of undress and/or close personal contacts. This suggests that potent adjustment areas will be those centering around sex, curiosity by others, clothing, and appearance. The study proposes to investigate the process of adjustment as it takes place within the hospital and throughout the first postoperative year. The personal nature of the problem is such that a variety of approaches and sources is to be used. These include: participant observation, interviews, check lists, and hospital records. As an exploratory investigation, the purpose is to search for hypotheses for subsequent testing.

In addition to formulating a general plan for collecting particular types of data from particular sets of respondents, research design needs also to deal with strategies for gaining access to the desired research site or sample of subjects. In this regard, sponsorship by persons holding key positions in the setting where the research is to be conducted is of singular importance. Without the support of sponsorship, the investigator may well find himself effectively blocked from implementing the study because he cannot gain entry to the social situation he wants to investigate. Kahn and Mann [33] suggest that successful field research in large, complex organizations depends on a methodology that provides for several important requirements, among which are multiple entry into the research site; contingent acceptance of the researcher(s) at different organizational levels; development of special liaison personnel; and access to the top person through both external and internal channels within the social structure of the organization.

Sponsorship in Health Research

In this matter of access to the field, cooperation from physicians is essential for anyone interested in studying people with health problems. The mastectomy study was developed and implemented as a joint project of the schools of nursing and medicine, a procedure that simplified the incorporation of private and nonprivate patients as part of the sample. This decision also meant that the investigator spent a considerable amount of time in conversation with members of the medical staff concerning the selection of hospitalized patients as subjects for investigation.

It is important that nurses not view this extremely important step of sponsorship as a matter of asking the doctor for permission to use "his patients." Rather, it is a means for conveying information about the study, for obtaining cooperation in its implementation, and for minimizing misunderstandings that might prevent its completion. The agreement to participate in any study involves contractual arrangements between the investigator and the subjects selected for the sample. However, it is important to be aware that access to the sample may well depend on the investigator's ability to negotiate successfully with individuals who have the power to block contact with the desired set of respondents. Thus an essential part of research design includes the identification of persons who have power to prevent negotiation with the desired sample of subjects [48] and, secondarily, the development of plans for gaining cooperation from them.

THE METHODOLOGY OF FIELD RESEARCH

As Pearsall [36] has pointed out, participant observation is a useful methodology for studying and thereby broadening scientific knowledge about human behavior within a given sociocultural or psychosocial context. Participant observation is characterized not as *a method* but rather as a combination of techniques and approaches for collecting information about a particular social group or organization and for using these data to create an analytic description of the human situation under study. By definition, participant observation refers to at least three phenomena: a role, a device for getting information, and a methodology for understanding human behavior within a given social context [36].

Types of Methods

The distinguishing characteristic of field research is that it involves the investigator in ongoing social interactions with the subjects under study for the purpose of making *direct observations* of events and incidents in progress. Because the investigator either cannot be present all of the time, or may be restricted from access to certain situations, or both, field studies must also rely on *indirect observations.* The latter are provided through interviews with key informants, namely, people who are present during critical incidents or are privy to special information not ordinarily available to an outsider. In studying death as a usual hospital event, for example, the field-workers were unable to be present during the entire period of time preceding a particular death. To piece together an account of the sequential nature of what took place, they had to make use of interviews with many different persons involved for a variety of reasons in the process of dying.

In addition to direct observation and interviews with informants, McCall and Simmons [34] indicate that the other techniques of document analysis, respondent interviews, and direct participation are typical and necessary if a thorough analytic description of any complex social organization is to be made. Zelditch [62] considers three field methods as primary: type I, participant-observations, referring to direct observation and participation in ongoing events; type II, informant-interviewing, referring to reports about events happening to people other than the informant; and type III, enumerations and samples referring to surveys and counting procedures. Clearly, the researcher in the field makes use of several different techniques of data collection for the purpose of obtaining different kinds of information to use in a comprehensive analysis of the social situation under examination.

To study the psychosocial meanings of being diabetic, for instance, the investigator utilized a variety of methods for collecting data about the effects of juvenile-onset diabetes mellitus on everyday patterns of living. The techniques included direct observations as participant observer in diabetic clinics and at diabetic camp; indirect observations through interviews with young diabetics and the members of their families; and utilization of hospital records for histories of the illness and assessments of medical control at different points in time.

Types of Data

Studies of human beings "in action" cannot depend on one type of data but rather are based on an effective pulling together of different types of information, each adding a dimension to the overall pattern of social structure and interaction. The study generally begins with a good deal of qualitative data that are obtained through descriptive accounts of particular events occurring at particular times to particular sets of people. The initial data usually appear as statements describing single properties of single or isolated events, and these descriptive incidents provide the building blocks out of which categories and complex configurations are formed. For example, Sudnow's [57] collection of incidents about hospital deaths provided systematic evidence to show that one section of the hospital was a critical place in which roughly three fourths of the deaths took place. The field data are systematically classified, enumerated, and compared as they are collected, and additional data are sought from the field to clarify that which appears to be missing or when new events make new data imperative for understanding.

The qualitative descriptions do not remain as such but eventually are combined into different classes of information. Zelditch [62] suggests that field observations can be combined into three broad classifications of information: type I, incidents and histories, referring to configurations of complex properties of either static or dynamic nature; type II, distributions and frequencies, referring to counts of given properties, activities, or events; and type III, generally known statuses and rules, referring to explicit statements made by participants or readily available through direct observation. Ultimately then, the researcher makes use of both quantitative and qualitative data in combination as he pursues the essential analysis.

By way of illustration, in the mastectomy study the women were initially classified into categories on the basis of such general statuses as age, marital status, and socioeconomic level. Healing of the incision was a property that eventually came to be used to subdivide the subjects into three distinct subgroups: those with satisfactory wound healing, those with delay in wound healing, and those who experienced manifest physical regression and death [41]. Of the 21 women, 6 fell into the first group; 13 were put into group two; and 2 made up the third classification. The final analysis showed that women in each of the three groups experienced a somewhat different history of encounters with other people, in great measure defined by the physical consequences subsequent to the mastectomy operation. Long before the final analysis could be done, however, the sample had to be located and decisions reached about the when, where, and how of gathering the necessary data from them.

Strategies in the Field

Once having chosen participant observation as the methodology, the investigator needs to be aware that the peculiarities of the field determine the approach and the procedures that can be used. In a practical sense, the investigator has to concern himself with such knotty matters as these: access to the field; selection of the participants to be sampled; consent to participate; development of protocols and instruments to guide the selection process; and the limitations that are imposed on the study by such concrete realities as time, money, and other people.

The living-in arrangement used by the cultural anthropologist for studying tribal cultures might be ideal for investigating how people live with chronic illness at home, but the approach is not realistic in urban societies for many reasons. The mastectomy study made use of a longitudinal design that produced a wealth of sensitive data. Such research is a costly enterprise, and it asks of those being studied (as well as of the researchers) a tremendous commitment of time, effort, and human energy [40]. In studying the impact of diabetes on diabetic adolescents and their families, a longitudinal approach was not practical, and a cross-sectional design was chosen as the alternative. Instead of following a small group of families over a period of time, e.g., a postoperative year, as was done in the mastectomy investigation, the data were collected only once from a number of families with different social characteristics and in different temporal stages of living with diabetes. In both investigations, the investigator had to decide how best to make contact with the subjects deemed to be suitable candidates for study.

The importance of sponsorship as a strategy for gaining access to the desired set of informants and respondents has already been discussed. Making contact with the subjects themselves requires careful planning that takes into account the special circumstances under which the initial meeting is to take place, as well as the investigator's expectations about the need for additional contacts. Not only must the researcher make some general decisions about what he wants to observe, and when and where, he must also concern himself with his own bearing and conduct so as to obtain the required information. The kinds of data that he obtains may well depend on the status that he chooses for introducing himself to the primary subjects and other people in the field of study. In this regard the nurse-researcher [10] may encounter both blessings and handicaps in the decision to reenter the field of the hospital in the openly acknowledged status of nurse. Some experiences taken from the mastectomy study serve to illustrate this point.

The mastectomy study depended on procedures and strategies to ensure contacts with the selected subjects not only during the period of hospitalization but also at selected intervals during the first year after the surgery. The study depended on data collection that was periodic rather than continuous and was done in different settings and under different sets of circumstances. It was concerned with subject matter that was emotionally delicate and sensitive in several different ways. Since success of the investigation depended on periodic contact with these women for a prolonged span of time, the maintenance of effective relationships depended on laying the proper groundwork while they were still hospitalized and, subsequently, on keeping avenues of communication open after they went home.

Early in planning, a decision was reached to have the data collected by a field-worker who made initial contact in the role of nurse assisting in the preoperative and postoperative care of the subjects but not assuming sole responsibility for it. During the preparatory phase of the study, certain key steps were taken. Hospital personnel and physicians were prepared for the advent of the nurse–field-workers, and a second nurse was selected to join the research project. The investigator engaged in some preliminary scanning observations that served as a guide for determining how best to contact the subjects and for judging the time periods that might be fruitful intervals for data collection. Some general decisions were made about the limits to be imposed on the uses of the role of nurse in direct patient care during the implementation of the study. The early experiences showed clearly that active involvement in certain activities of nursing precluded effective functioning in the primary role of observer. Hence a decision was made [38] to limit the periods of observation to those which made few demands on the technical and medical observation skills of the nurse. In effect, an effort was made to reduce the opportunity for role conflict in the nurse-researcher who was functioning as participant-as-observer so that data collection could assume priority over nursing care activities.

In retrospect, the success of maintaining contact with the women for the full span of time (with only one voluntary dropout) may well be tied to the choice of making an entree in the active role of nurse. In a sense, the provision of direct care by the researcher created a situation in which the women may have felt the need to reciprocate by continuing as subjects in the study [60]. That is, the reciprocal nature of the relationship between observer and observed may well have been strengthened by the act of care itself. There are serious problems to be faced in assuming the dual roles of nurse and researcher, however, and the complexities of the participant-as-observer are considered later. It is perhaps well to note at this point that the researcher's selection of a particular social position – in this case, nurse – sets limiting conditions on the data that are available to him. The identification of any investigator's status in the field [58] influences the image that is formed in the minds of the respondents and determines the settings that are made available to him.

Sampling Procedures

The selection of informants and respondents is guided by information obtained during the preliminary stages of the research. The study of diabetic adolescents emerged out of a large comparative investigation of the psychosocial meanings of chronic disease in adolescence. The decision to center attention on diabetes mellitus came after a year of participant observation in pediatric clinics providing services for children with three long-term diseases: cystic fibrosis, diabetes mellitus, and bronchial asthma. Analysis of the early data showed that reactions to chronic disease were affected by whether or not the disease and treatment were explicitly visible to ordinary people, and this observation led to the choice of social visibility as a central concept for organizing the study and analyzing the meaning of chronicity [45] to young people. The next requirement was selection of one disease for intensive investigation.

Although infrequently mentioned in the literature, decisions about sampling are often governed by practical realities as well as theoretical considerations. The choice of studying diabetic families was essentially guided by both. With respect to matters of practicality, families accustomed to an atmosphere of open conversation about the disease (as was found with diabetes) were seen as being receptive to being studied *as a whole.* In contrast, families in which a closed pattern of talk had been observed (as in the case of cystic fibrosis) were perceived as not too amenable to participation in total family interviewing [5]. Hence the choice of diabetes was seen as a relatively easy way of making a transition to the next phase of the study.

The selection of cases in the diabetes study was also based on the concept of theoretical sampling, and the comparison groups were selected for their relevance to the formulation of categories basic to development of substantive theory. Unlike statistical sampling in which the groups to be compared are defined and delimited in advance, theoretical sampling [24] allows for a broad selection of groups to maximize the comparative value of the data. Rather than to control for differences, the groups are chosen *because* of their differences in properties.

In the diabetes study, the two central comparison groups were families and young diabetics [46]. Four criteria were used for selecting different types of families: socioeconomic status; number of parents living in the household; number of diabetics living in the home; and years since the onset of diabetes. The criteria used for choosing the young diabetics were age, sex, and age at onset of diabetes. It is important to note that the criteria were not decided in advance but rather were selected as the study was in progress. This approach to sampling in no way means that groups are chosen haphazardly. Rather, it means that the reasons for selecting comparison groups in this type of study [24] are different from the reasons for selecting particular groups in studies that utilize statistical sampling procedures.

Decisions about the desired characteristics of the sample of respondents may be relatively simple. The actual collection of the data tends to be a far more difficult and often messy process involving the management of time and effective negotiation with individuals and groups of individuals. Making contact with the desired set of respondents and informants in the field was facilitated in the mastectomy study by the decision to enter in the social position of nurse. However, a good deal of time and effort had to be devoted to establishing effective working relationships with key persons in the hospital system so that potential subjects were made known to the project staff. First contacts with potential candidates were made on the evening prior to surgery, and sometimes more than one person was scheduled for breast surgery on the following day. The decision to see all women facing breast surgery meant that in addition to the presurgery hours spent with the 21 women who comprised the final sample, the investigators also collected data from 27 other women who underwent breast biopsies but did not become subjects for the follow-up study. This matter of collecting extraneous data is to be expected in field research until the analysis reaches a point of focus. Strauss et al. [56] have described in some detail the process of moving from a broad and generalized perspective in the field to a final phase of pinpointing hypotheses through deliberate, controlled inquiry and observation.

In the mastectomy study, the investigator's familiarity with the setting of the hospital served to facilitate the process of locating and holding the sample chosen for study. Such an opportunity is not generally available in unfamiliar settings where the fieldworker has to feel his way into a new social situation while at the same time he is defining and finding his sample [32]. Indeed, the characteristics of the social context may be such as to make negotiation with the desired respondents a complicated and sometimes unsuccessful enterprise.

During the diabetes study, for example, the opportunity for face-to-face contacts with the subjects in the chosen sample was not always possible, as had been true in the mastectomy investigation. Thus negotiation for participation became complicated by social distance in certain cases. Initial conversations with five of the families took place during their visits to an outpatient department, but four of the families were approached initially by telephone. The investigator preferred face-to-face contact for negotiation because of the broader range of interactional cues that it would make available, but telephone conversation per se did not appear to be a major deterrent to successful negotiation. It did, however, place the investigator in a disadvantaged position for pursuing negotiations that were tentative, and it placed those who were interested in refusal in a position of considerable power [1].

The approach to the young diabetic and his parent was one of asking for help, and the point was made that participation in the project was "not going to help you personally." Negotiation with the young people met with no major obstacles, nor were problems encountered with seven of the parents. In two of the families, efforts to obtain total family interviewing were effectively blocked by the mothers, and only part of the family was available for interview. Two additional families, both of which were working class, were approached, but negotiation with the parents was unsuccessful. This type of resistance to participation in clinical research by working-class parents, notably fathers, has also been reported by other investigators [3]. The point is that field-workers, like other investigators, can encounter serious difficulties in obtaining an adequate and complete sample of respondents and informants because of particular beliefs and practices over which the researcher has no control.

Guidelines and Protocols

The researcher in the field constantly makes choices and decisions that limit the data in some fashion. To ensure that his data are collected systematically, the field-worker uses a variety of protocols and instruments to guide the collection procedures. As has already been noted, the selection of the sample is guided by protocols developed during the preliminary phases of the study. Other kinds of guidelines are formulated as the study progresses to assist the observer in keeping his inquiry systematic and in guarding against bias of various kinds. The field-worker needs to be aware that bias is a universal phenomenon and that procedures need to be developed for identifying bias that can distort observations and limit the validity of the data [53].

The matter of time and timing cannot be underestimated in field research. Planning needs to take account of the reality of regular as well as unusual events to be encountered. The timing of observations during the implementation of the mastectomy project was affected by several considerations. There was need to establish a systematic pattern of observation for use within the hospital and, at the same time, to develop a schedule for home visits at specified time intervals. The purpose of the schedule was to ensure that each subject would be observed on a more or less regular basis, to enable the field-workers to follow the temporal order of events systematically, and to provide opportunity for locating points of similarity and divergence in the experience of the subjects.

While the women were hospitalized, the researchers maintained daily contact with them for two reasons: The contact paved the way for a request to continue observations at home, and it provided an opportunity to obtain the story of events preceding the surgery and to make direct observations of contacts with hospital personnel. Other observation periods were selected to permit opportunity to talk with members of the family or to be present when significant activities took place. An example of the latter category is the first dressing change.

Time management was easier to handle within the setting of the hospital where the nurse–field-worker had control over the situation than it was following discharge from the hospital. At this point the women could delay or refuse to have visits at home. Home contacts with the subjects were planned to occur at relatively frequent intervals during the first six months because this period was perceived as critical for them. In practice, the scheduling of these interviews became flexible rather than rigid to accommodate to the social contingencies of the women and their families. In a sense, the worker in the field has to be willing to modify his predetermined design and to collect the data as it is made available to him by the respondents.

The importance of timing and time requires a certain amount of flexibility and openness from the researcher. He must be able to modify his schedule of activities to accommodate to new events and unexpected occurrences in the ongoing process of data collection. During the implementation of the mastectomy study, the matter of timing was a precarious venture and highly unpredictable. Implementation of the project required the establishment of some kind of balanced approach to the maintenance of home visits and observation periods in the hospital. Sometimes the pressures on the observers were intense, as happened when three women were hospitalized at the same time.

Since timing of observations is related to what is deemed relevant to observe, the data collected during the early phases of fieldwork serve an important function. These data provide direction for deciding which areas are sufficiently important to pursue in detail during the more focused period of data collection. During the mastectomy study, the substance of the preliminary observations served as a guide for deciding what was important to these women. For example, the appearance of the incision was a shocking experience for most of them. Thus conversation about the incision was incorporated into each of the home interviews, to ascertain whether their reactions changed and how they coped with any problems associated with the incision as time went by.

Initially, the participant observer engages in interviews that tend to be informal and somewhat generalized in focus. As particular substantive areas are identified, he uses the ongoing analysis of data to develop guidelines and direction for focused interviews for the purpose of obtaining specific data about these selected areas of concern. Thus the first home interview in the mastectomy study covered three broad areas: a picture of what had happened since the woman left the hospital; a picture of how the woman felt between the time of knowing surgery was scheduled and the postsurgery period; and a picture of how she viewed the period of hospitalization. The schedules for subsequent interviews covered some of the same general areas but were modified to incorporate other areas of interest chosen as a result of the ongoing analysis of new data.

The instruments developed to guide the collection of the data are dependent on the types of data required and the variety of respondents involved. Where a heterogeneous sample of subjects is to be used, the development of appropriate tools can be complicated and time-consuming. In planning for the study of diabetic adolescents and their families, for instance, a decision was made to interview entire families on the assumption that data from all members of the household would give a more valid image of the social meanings of diabetes than could be obtained by restricting the interviews to parents and diabetic child. The substantive areas to be investigated in detail came from analysis of data obtained through observations and interviews with 16 partial families in a pediatric diabetic clinic. Initially, a general guide was developed and utilized for interviews with one family, but one protocol was found to be inadequate for obtaining differences in perspective associated with differences in status. Subsequently, separate interview schedules were developed for use with the three types of informants, namely, the principal subjects, the parents, and the siblings.

The Interview as Negotiation

The format for the interview used in the diabetes study would probably be classified as the nonschedule, standardized type, which, according to Richardson, Dohrenwend, and Klein [48], is most appropriate for dealing with sensitive topics where the respondents are heterogeneous. The schedule was set up to include topics that were basic to each interview, but the interviewer was free to word questions so that they were understandable to each respondent. The approach also allows for a shift in sequence of topics if such a change is in keeping with the readiness and mood of the interviewee. In actual practice, the interviews combined a nonstandardized approach with a standardized and semistructured format, a procedure made possible because the investigator in charge of the study was conducting all of the interviews and was completely familiar with its conceptual framework. In this case, standardization refers to the *classes of information* being sought rather than to the employment of identically worded questions with each respondent.

Each interview can perhaps best be described as a continuous flow of negotiation involving both participants in a bargaining process. In implementing the diabetes study, the negotiation required a sensitivity to the complexity of social relationships within each of the families. The bargaining process whereby information was exchanged was heavily dependent on the investigator's flexibility, both in creating an atmosphere conducive to open discussion and in shifting easily from role to role as the occasion demanded.

The interviews were easiest to perform when the respondents were women, and the investigator (also a woman) could identify readily with the roles they were playing and describing. The process of bargaining was more of an effort when the respondents were children, especially young ones who easily shifted from role of subject to role of child without benefit of politeness or decorum. The strategies used were basically aimed at obtaining information about the meaning of diabetes within the respondent's frame of reference; hence it was necessary to pay almost constant attention to the two interacting factors of verbal messages and nonverbal cues [46]. The latter requirement results in interviewing that is characteristically high in stress for the interviewer.

As has been pointed out by a number of astute observers [11, 20, 52], the meaning of any data collected by man interacting with man must take account of the reality that the investigator relies on commonsense knowledge and everyday language when he selectively notices certain events and makes certain choices about their relevance, including a determination that they are "measurements" of some kind. Stated in somewhat different terms, the process of interviewing involves human beings with all of their idiosyncratic, situational, and cultural variations coming into play, so that bias and selective interpretation are built-in features [31].

Procedures for Data Recording

Since the participant observer collects data under a variety of social and cultural conditions, he needs to plan for the systematic recording of these data so as to take into account the many distortions of bias and selective perception that are in operation. In investigations that center around the psychosocial meanings of death, systematic record-keeping is a tremendously important process in that researcher and researched alike tend easily to be caught up in unresolved feelings about death and dying. In fact, the project director of any study concerned with emotion-laden subject matter must be prepared to offer special training to the field investigators that he uses and to develop mechanisms for providing ongoing support to them while they are in process of collecting the data [44].

The problem of bias is more readily available for identification when the investigator establishes a systematic method for the recording of data, including the incorporation of his own reactions to events in the field as well as actions that he may take. The most common recording method used by researchers in the field is record-keeping in the form of a field journal or daily log in which observations are regularly jotted down, along with interpretations of what has been observed. So that the information can be readily understood at a later point in time, the investigator usually develops a code whereby he can separate the observations from the interpretations. Thus Strauss et al. [56] made use of different notational conventions to differentiate recorded information that was exact recall from that which was uncertain or only partially remembered.

In essence, the participant observer needs to devise a way whereby he can later make sense out of the different types of data that he records in his notes. He must also develop the habit of writing up his notes on a systematic basis during the period of data collection. Though the practice of self-discipline in record-keeping may well interfere with his social life for a limited period of time, it can make a fundamental difference in the quality of research that is produced. The intricacies of observation, maintenance of records, and analysis of what is happening during the early days in the field have been clearly and usefully documented by Geer [21].

Because the researcher in the field is seldom in position to take notes while he is engaged in conversation with his informants, he usually has to develop ways of taking mental notes. That is, he learns to create reminders in his thoughts to serve as cues when he begins to record his data later in the day. At first, the task may appear impossible, and the new investigator tends to feel overwhelmed by the vast amount of information available to him. With practice, the investigator can increase both the amount and the accuracy of his observations. A notebook kept in the pocket can often be useful for jotting down key phrases as reminders for later transcription. A checklist may also be used, so that the fieldworker can, from time to time, see whether or not his own blind spots are causing him to omit certain kinds of observations. Conferences with a consultant are especially helpful in identifying the problem areas of missing data, personal reactions, and distortions in observation. Effective use of such conferences can be facilitated if written field notes are available to serve as a focus for discussion. A tape recording of conferences can also be helpful as a form of data-retrieval. If transcribed, these notes provide another source of data for analysis.

Checks on the validity and reliability of observations are more readily available in research in which a team of investigators monitor and challenge the others' observations. In research performed by a single investigator, the importance of disciplined recording of all observations, reactions, and interpretations is crucial. Only thus can the contaminating effects of personal distortion and limitation of observation be identified clearly and used in the analysis. To explain the meaning of his data, the investigator needs to be sure that he systematically keeps account not only of what he observes but also of the structural conditions under which the observations were made [12].

It is clear that observations can be recorded in great detail when mechanical methods such as videotape or audiotape recordings are used. Such procedures increase the costs of research tremendously, and they are often not practical approaches for investigations in the field. They can, however, be extremely useful for collecting information under selected sets of circumstances. For example, the five home interviews conducted as part of the mastectomy study were all recorded on audiotape for later transcription. These recordings produced a wealth of data that could not have been detailed through the maintenance of written field journals. They also produced considerable turnover in the project's secretarial staff because the experiences being transcribed from the tapes triggered reactions of depression and personal identification. The time required to transcribe tape recordings slows the process of analysis, and the process can be slowed even more when the recordings describe events that cause the staff members concerned to become deeply involved emotionally. These kinds of problems are to be anticipated in any research concerned with the phenomenon of human death.

Limitations of the Data

Anyone engaged in social research needs to be aware that his personal characteristics influence and limit the kinds of data that he obtains. For example, the information used in the mastectomy study was all collected by women. Had the investigators been men, it is probable that a somewhat different set of findings might have been reported. In doing research about death and related matters, the investigator's age, sex, appearance, and identified status all affect what other people will consider appropriate to tell or not to tell him.

In addition to personal characteristics, the data are also limited by the structural conditions of the setting in which data collection takes place. When collecting information about the experiences of young diabetics at summer camp, for instance, the investigator did not have direct access to the camp areas housing the boys and thus had to rely on indirect observations provided through conversations with the male counselors. Stated generally, there are limitations on the data imposed by lack of access to certain types of events and activities. There are also other structural conditions that limit the information in various ways. For example, the sequence of interviews with members of a given group, such as families with diabetic members, determines which information will be brought to the investigator's attention first. Moreover, failure to make contact with a key person in the social situation under study can create a serious gap in the data available for analysis.

The field-worker does not have at his beck and call all possible data about the group that he is studying. Thus he needs to understand that the validity and reliability of his reported findings are strengthened to the extent that he utilizes multiple resources for his data, establishes reasonable methods for checking on his actions and observations, and reports his methods and interpretations with integrity. McCall [34] suggests that the key to quality control in participant observation comes through the use of multiple indicants to support a given fact and insistence on a high degree of consistency among these various indicants.

The matter of being sensitive to personal reactions and responses is of critical importance in research about death and dying. The topic is tension-producing for human beings in general, and researchers are not exempt from these kinds of reactions and responses. Investigators cannot always anticipate what is likely to happen to them when they start talking with other people about death and dying. This phenomenon was clearly brought home during the implementation of the mastectomy study when the nurse-researchers were brought face to face with their personal feelings about cancer and mastectomy [39, 40]. The experience showed clearly that research about death must be planned to incorporate usable mechanisms for helping the investigators to cope with intense emotional reactions to the data they are in process of collecting.

Data Analysis and Interpretation

All methods in science involve a relationship between the investigator and the subject matter being considered. Where human behavior is at issue, the relationship is exceedingly complex in that researcher and subjects alike create the data through interactions that meet their personal and collective needs as human beings [50]. It is increasingly evident that the crucial instrument for measurement and assessment in all research is the investigator himself, and that criteria of validity, reliability, and objectivity are established relative to a chosen frame of reference and are affected by the characteristics of the available data [9]. When the data to be used are primarily qualitative in nature, the researcher faces the complex task of developing procedures whereby he can systematically code, index, and compare rather large amounts of uneven information.

To some extent the purpose of the study determines the specifics of the approach chosen for analysis. Becker and Geer [2] devised a method whereby qualitative data are used to "constitute proof" for given propositions through a series of coding, analyzing, and checking operations. For example, to pinpoint student perspectives on proper nurse behaviors in the face of death, the investigator systematically reviewed all descriptive anecdotes, identified viewpoints offered by students or indicated by their behaviors, checked the frequency of the viewpoints in the available data, looked for negative cases, and compared the viewpoints by class for changes over time [43].

Berelson [6] suggested that qualitative data can be translated into quantitative data and then subjected to a strict content analysis. To illustrate this technique, a historical investigation of professional interest in death, as reflected in publication, would mean systematic study of all articles and books dealing with death to identify the frequencies and distributions of major themes or concepts presented.

When qualitative data are used for theory development, Glaser [22] proposed an ongoing method of explicit coding and comparative analysis that is continuous. Using this method, the investigator coded the diabetes study data as they were collected and used the categories to formulate ideas about a theory of chronicity [45]. No matter whether the purpose be hypothesis testing or theory building, the investigator needs to develop systematic ways of handling the data so that it can be subjected to the logic of analytic induction [49].

To some extent, ongoing analysis of the data is procedurally built into the process of participant observation. As the study progresses, however, the investigator develops specific guidelines to help him complete the final analysis. Prior to this time, he needs to find ways of keeping records of ideas that come to mind, and one approach is through the systematic writing of memos that are filed for future reference. Another approach is that of coding the categorized data on cards that can be cross-indexed in a variety of ways.

Sometime later, the investigator develops analytic protocols to assist him in further indexing and comparing the data. To complete the diabetes study, for example, three analytic schedules were devised. The first was designed for making comparisons about the social processes whereby families learn to live with diabetes. The second was devised to consider the present meaning of disease and treatment for each family. The third was formulated using the concepts of status passage and role identity as theoretical underpinnings to provide guidelines for clarifying the process whereby young diabetics learn what it means to be diabetic [46].

The analysis itself usually takes place by phases and stages. In fact, the "emergent nature" of data analysis is a phrase that seems to characterize best the process whereby conceptual categories are formulated and conceptual ties are identified. When the diabetic study was in process of completion, the analytic procedures moved simultaneously in two directions. Each family was analyzed as a unit, while at the same time there was a comparative analysis with all the other families. The coding and intrafamily comparisons resulted in two analytic memos for each set of interviews, one dealing with the process of change and the other focused on the present state of affairs within the family. The data for each of the young diabetics were analyzed within the social context of his family relationships, and they were also subjected to cross-comparisons with other diabetic subjects. The final report of the study was concerned with three components of analysis: identification of the sequence and stages whereby parents come to function as agents of diabetic treatment; differentiation of family patterns of adaptation to diabetes; and specification of the stages by which a diabetic identity is formed. The final report also contained a clear statement of the limitations of the reported findings.

Notwithstanding the importance of protocols and procedures to guide the handling of the data, the crux of analysis lies in the formulation of new insights and conceptualizations about the phenomenon being studied. Analysis of the mastectomy data provided rich data to show how the diagnosis of cancer functions as a stigmatizing influence in the lives of those who bear the disease [42]. Investigating the process whereby patients with serious metabolic conditions deal with the life stresses of uncertainty and danger, Fox observed that patterned humor about death and other serious concerns that these patients shared in common served a tension-releasing function for them in their social life on a research ward [18]. A published report of the latter study contains a cogent and interesting description of the process whereby the investigator first became aware of the uses of "grim humor" and then went about the business of locating evidence to verify the validity of the observations.

Not uncommonly, insight into the meanings of a set of findings may not appear immediately but may even come to mind, sometimes quite unexpectedly, long after the investigation has been formally completed. More than that, the findings of one study often serve as the triggering mechanism for another. Sometimes they may create an opportunity for the investigator to join a research team interested in studying a similar or related problem. The latter event occurred to me when the research about mastectomy provided entree into a team investigation of dying patients and hospital personnel [23, 25, 43]. The sequential nature of research is manifest in a kind of chain reaction whereby the outcomes of one investigation contribute directly to the evolution of many others.

THE ROLE OF PARTICIPANT OBSERVER

As was certainly true in the mastectomy study, utilization of the nurse role was a useful means for making contact with the subjects chosen for study. There were several types of problems, however, that were associated with this choice. The first had to do with the competency of the observer with respect to selection of appropriate content, accuracy in noting and in recording, and recognition of personal bias. The experience brought clearly to mind the selective perceptions of nurses in the hospital and the interfering effect of these perceptions on "seeing" events in other kinds of ways. In effect, the observations within the hospital required a retraining of focus so that the field-worker could view the scene less as a nurse and more as an observer of social interaction.

Associated with this data-gathering process were other kinds of difficulties attendant on being identified in the role of nurse. The problem of deception in relationships with patients and with staff had to be handled by each field-worker in her own way. The importance of protecting informants and keeping the data confidential meant that talk about the study was confined to project staff members or to selected individuals who could be trusted. This decision meant that the researchers had to control their interactions with physicians and nurses and thereby assume a new and different role with colleagues. There were moments when each field-worker thought of herself as a traitor.

In the continuing role of observer, the field-workers encountered serious personal difficulties in maintaining their contacts with the subjects, primarily because of the emotional tensions associated with breast loss and cancer. Loss of a breast and its associated sexual identification are not topics easily discussed, nor is the prospect of dying from cancer. Thus the investigators faced the task of encouraging talk about two relatively taboo topics made additionally troublesome to the interviewers because they were also women. In fact, one of the major difficulties throughout the study was a tendency to identify personally with the problems these women faced [39].

The Observer as Nurse

A second problem arose because the field-workers were identified as nurses by the women participants as well as by others in the setting, and they faced certain difficulties associated with this identification. The principal dilemma centered around decisions concerning when it was appropriate to behave as a nurse and when it was not. These decisions were important because patient care activity could interfere with or influence the field-worker's principal task, which was to gather relevant data.

In the hospital, one of the critical difficulties for the nurse in the position of participant-as-observer has to do with setting limits on active participation as a nurse. The decision to limit activity as a nurse may be easier to state than to put into action, because the nurse who is also observer eventually comes face to face with concrete problems that demand a choice between being a nurse and being an observer. The problem may even be accentuated if the nurse-researcher decides that the nursing staff is not taking care of the problem in question. During the implementation of the mastectomy study, for example, detachment from active involvement with a woman who resisted arm exercises was difficult to maintain, and especially so when a colleague in the school of nursing questioned the field-worker's responsibilities in this matter. This illustration points to two difficulties nurses are prone to face: feelings of guilt for failing to implement action that is viewed as a nursing responsibility, and implied criticism from other nurses for failure to be a "good nurse."

Physical care posed fewer problems than did conversations with patients, primarily because decisions governing the latter issue could not always be clear and concise. Since part of a nurse's function is to provide information to patients, the cutoff point for this activity was difficult to establish. In part, the problem arose during the mastectomy study because of the close and continuous investigator-subject relationship that was required to facilitate data collection. This requirement removed many of the protective devices nurses have available to protect them from knowing what is happening to patients and from personal involvement in patients' lives.

Perhaps the best way to illustrate the difficulty is to describe a specific incident that took place while the study was in progress. Early analysis of the data showed that the women were given very little information about what to expect after leaving the hospital and what to do in an emergency. The nurse–field-worker who had joined the project began to coach the new subjects about these matters until the project director pointed out that one purpose of the study was to understand how the hospital experience affected their lives. The field-worker's responsibility was to note what was happening but not to intervene to provide that which was missing. Because withholding of care – in this instance the giving of information – is considered *poor nursing*, to behave in such a way produces conflict in the nurse who defines her self-expectations in terms of the provision of care. The nurse–field-worker who can accept the notion that responsibility for patient care rests with the hospital staff and not with her alone can more comfortably live with herself when she encounters patient care that appears inadequate in her eyes.

Although the field-workers functioned as nurses in the hospital, they were not officially in this capacity during interviews in the subjects' homes. They did not leave the nurse identity behind, however, and several important problems were encountered. For one thing, the women knew them as nurses and treated them as knowledgeable authorities to whom they could turn for answers to their medical questions. These questions were of two general types: those pertaining to breast cancer in general and those pertaining to their personal well-being. Both gave the field-workers trouble.

The women were freer to ask questions of the researchers than of their physicians, and to avoid this problem the researchers told the women that they were not privileged to give this kind of information. The observers found the situation a difficult one, and especially so when they became aware that a woman had been given few details about her true condition and was seeking some answers. Moreover, the field-workers experienced considerable difficulty in giving the women straightforward information about breast cancer, yet they were often faced with such inquiries [40].

Conversations with the women required a delicate balance between nurse-to-patient talk and woman-to-woman talk. The interviews were difficult to carry on because some of the content roused tension in both interviewer and respondent. What took place during these conversations was influenced by a variety of factors, including differences in age, vocabulary, marital status, ethnicity, and social class. The field-workers had to be ready to deal with efforts to block the conversation and to be prepared for the direct rebuff. As they learned through experience, conversation about emotionally disturbing matters can provoke strong emotional responses, which may be difficult to understand if one is not expecting them.

As the study continued, the analysis of data suggested strongly that the educational experience of becoming a nurse has not contained adequate preparation for coping well with this kind of conversation with patients. The nurse has been taught that nurses avoid undue familiarity with patients, and she has developed techniques for maintaining conversational detachment from them. To achieve the valued professional goal of controlling public display of emotions, she has learned strategies for avoiding topics that may be difficult to handle. Much of her training has been directed toward the management of conversation to achieve certain therapeutic goals deemed important by medical and nursing authority. The process of education has encouraged a stereotyped pattern of interacting with patients, and the nurse is likely to find the situation difficult when the conversational stance expected is not governed by explicit rules. In a sense, the experience as practitioner has ill-prepared the nurse for fieldwork as a technique for research.

The nurse who uses the methodology of participant observation to investigate patient-focused problems is vulnerable on yet another score. She may choose problems which bring her face to face with the full impact of pain, sorrow, emptiness, and want, but without the protection of institutionalized operations and tactics which formerly barred her from this kind of exposure. In a setting which deprives her of the well-established privilege of using her hands to provide physical comfort, the nurse may find herself ill at ease and unable to listen when difficult subjects are under discussion. When confronted with these problems, she may well find herself responding to the tension by assuming a "taking care of" role with the respondents and of being available to them in a way that is beyond that expected by the study and appropriate to its execution. These difficulties can probably not be completely avoided by nurses. They can be attenuated if psychiatric counseling and other kinds of consultation are available (as needed) to assist the nurse in understanding what is taking place.

The problems of role conflict are undoubtedly not unique to nurses but would take place for any field-worker who returns to a familiar place of work and attempts to utilize an old status in a new way. The difficulties can be particularly acute for nurses, however, when they attempt to investigate problems that have strong emotional ties with their previously established identity as nurse.

Social Isolation and Bias

The decision to participate actively as a nurse-observer in the hospital or other clinical facility sets in motion an ongoing process requiring that the observer make frequent choices about when and when not to engage in the normal and usual activities expected of nurses in that setting. In a sense, the observer-nurse has to establish the position of a nurse participating in patient care without assuming complete management of it. Such activity requires a delicate balancing of professional relationships.

During the implementation of the mastectomy study, the nurse—field-workers assisted the physicians with a variety of procedures and engaged in verbal exchanges with them, but the participation was initiated for the purpose of collecting data. The observers made no effort to participate in all such incidents that they encountered. In like manner, they assumed responsibility for certain nursing tasks and discussed nursing care problems with other nurses, but they did not take complete charge of the care provided. Initially, the observers were viewed with doubt, as though the staff wondered, "What do you *really* want?" As the work was shared, suspicion diminished, and the staff became accustomed to the observers' presence. The field-workers, however, had to learn to live with a sense of isolation from the staff. As observers, they could not truly be part of the staff's experience as a collectivity, nor could the staff permit this to happen.

One danger of this marginal position is that it makes for a concentrated exposure to the patient's viewpoint and can produce an identification so forceful that the behavior of the staff may be perceived completely from this bias and with little understanding of their perspectives and pressures. Such overidentification may, for example, cause the observer to intervene with the physician in a way that triggers antagonism and misunderstanding. An incident of this type may effectively block future communication. Evidence obtained in the mastectomy study showed that the physician was extremely sensitive to comments by others when a patient's prognosis was poor and he could offer little help. Yet under the same circumstances the observer was likely to be captured in her own set of tensions and to interact in a manner that provoked anger.

Since the bias of the field-worker influences both the reporting and the recording of observations, notes kept during such periods will carry the emotional tone of the observer's reactions. However, the investigator may well find that at a later point in time, when detachment has replaced emotional involvement, these notes can be perused from the viewpoint of *observer* and *reporter* rather than from the involved perspective of the *participant* who made them. Anyone who investigates human death and dying is bound to encounter incidents that trigger strong emotional reactions. He needs to be aware that these events are likely to occur and to view them as important data to be systematically recorded, analyzed, and interpreted.

ETHICS IN RESEARCH ABOUT DEATH

The decision to participate in research using the active role of professional nursing practitioner requires that explicit attention be given to the issue of intervention on behalf of the patient and the conditions under which intervention would be mandatory. The nurse so engaged needs to be aware of and to practice standards of conduct that are recognized in the law for the protection of persons against unusual risks of harm [28]. In this regard, the nurse would be advised to use as a guideline the standards and orders regularly used by the nursing staffs offering services to patients in the community and institution where the study is being done. It seems clear that in an extreme emergency, when no physician is readily available and relief of a critical state must be obtained rapidly [29], the nurse would be expected to assist the patient toward improvement in his condition.

Despite the availability of general guidelines and ethical codes for professional practice, the decisions in the field do not always take place under circumstances in which the proper choice can be clearly and easily identified. For as Ellis [14] has noted, although the primary ethic for nursing is the welfare of the patient, how best to provide for that welfare is generally a matter of judgment. Moreover, the issue of intervention on behalf of the patient is complicated and often uncertain when the situation requiring judgment from the nurse involves the death or possible death of a patient. As Savard [51] has noted, to date there has been no clearly established set of principles and guidelines to assist paramedical health professionals in defining their moral and ethical responsibilities towards patients who are also subjects in clinical research. Notwithstanding this lack, the nurse who chooses to investigate human experiences with death and dying may well encounter situations that raise moral and legal questions and concerns. Easy solutions to such problems may be hard to find.

Decisions to Intervene

As was indicated earlier, decisions about disclosure of medical information was one problem encountered while the data were collected for the mastectomy study. Another difficulty arose when concern about the patient's need for medical care became a pressing issue for the nurse-observer. The latter problem asserted itself when the question of suicide was raised, or when the woman's physical condition so distressed the nurse that she felt compelled to do something about it. Problems of this sort were discussed with the surgeon co-investigator, whose principal function in the study was to provide consultation about just such matters when they appeared. Access to this form of consultation was an important mechanism for coping with difficult problems that called for medical advice and that suggested the need for outside intervention. Any nurse using fieldwork to investigate problems about patients and patient care might expect to encounter serious dilemmas that can best be resolved with the help of medical or other professional opinion. To be maximally effective and useful, the mechanism for consultation needs to be built into the basic design of the research.

Protection of Human Rights

The plan for the study needs also to take account of the confidential nature of data provided by human subjects and to provide the means whereby participants are informed about the general purposes for which the research is being done. The position taken here is that research about human behavior is a cooperative enterprise that involves collaboration between the investigator and the persons being studied [35]. Such being the case, the investigator recognizes the importance of providing for informed consent both at the formal level of agreement between researcher and researched and at the informal level of transient contact with other persons encountered while the study is in progress.

The function of informed consent is to describe the study in enough detail that the participant has some understanding of what the research is about and is offered the option of nonparticipation if he so chooses. In a very real sense, the investigator and the investigated enter into a contract whereby information is shared on the assumption that it will not be used by the researcher in a way that is harmful or hurtful. The ethics of research suggest that this agreement places a heavy burden of responsibility on the researcher to respect the information that is made available to him. This being the case, the researcher who is studying a subject as sensitive and tension-producing as death needs to take every precaution to maintain the records of the study and the data itself in a location that is protected from easy access by others.

The ethical issues associated with informed consent and confidentiality of the data are extremely complex when children are used as subjects for research [55]. Especially is this the case when the problem being studied deals with sensitive subjects such as death or involves the entire family as participants. Making arrangements for participation in the diabetes study, for example, required that two agreements had to be negotiated, one with the young diabetic and the other with his parents. Negotiation for consent meant offering an explanation that was motivationally stimulating to each. It also meant obtaining specific agreements as to time, place, and willingness to participate.

To guard against invasion of privacy, the agreement was made that information obtained from the interview with each person living in the household would not be shared with other members of the family. The investigator took the position that it would have been a deliberate misrepresentation to utilize privileged information from one interview to enter the private domain of another member of the family, unless an invitation to do so was extended by that person himself [15]. As a result of this choice, certain of the data were more limited in detail than was desirable for completeness of understanding. Like the ethics of clinical practice, the ethics of research involving human beings [61] sometimes require that the investigator give up access to certain data out of respect for the privacy of the individual. The investigator also has responsibility to see that other staff members employed to work on the study clearly understand the confidential nature of their work.

Reports of Findings

Just as the investigator carries moral obligations to protect the privacy of human beings who choose to participate in research with him, so also does he have an obligation to make his findings known through clear and detailed publication [26]. Protecting the identity of individual informants is an accepted ethical standard in research, and published reports often make use of pseudonyms and other devices to minimize the identification of people and places. In practice, the protection of identity may not be a simple matter, as happens when the group being studied is small or so well known that publication is equivalent to open disclosure. Recently, a suggestion was made that certain types of social problems might properly be studied without the promise of confidentiality, but even here, no claim is made that such an approach should be common practice in behavioral research [47].

Publication of sensitive findings can pose special difficulties if the investigator is concerned that an open report of results might be injurious to the persons who provided the data. Sometimes a preliminary report of the findings may be presented to groups of respondents to provide them opportunity to react to the results prior to publication. Sometimes the timing of publication may be all that is necessary to avoid unpleasant reaction, and a reasonable interval before offering a public report will allow opportunity for the findings to be tempered by time. Often, the investigator's concerns are groundless, and published reports may even be welcomed. He must be aware, however, that articles reporting on sensitive and delicate matters can trigger unexpected and sometimes unpleasant responses among colleagues and other professional groups as well as among laymen [19]. A judicious and careful choice of words is always of importance in the presentation of research of this type.

KNOWLEDGE AND HUMAN AFFAIRS

Few ready-made solutions exist for the kinds of problems and issues that research about death produces for the person interested in expanding knowledge about the meaning of death in human affairs. Yet knowledge about the intricate social and personal nature of dying can probably best be gained by employing the methodology of participant observation to full advantage. The complexities and intricacies of using the position of nurse to study the psychosocial effects of life-threatening disease have been described in some detail. The demanding and rigorous requirements of investigations about sensitive human experiences such as these need to be recognized in advance and procedures built into the research process for maintaining a systematic and disciplined approach in the face of personal involvements of several kinds. If one purpose of behavioral research is to provide objective and analytic description about highly subjective human experience, the difficulties of the task cannot be underestimated.

ACKNOWLEDGMENTS

The study of adjustment following mastectomy was supported by a grant (M-5495) from the National Institute of Mental Health, United States Public Health Service, and was conducted through the University of California at Los Angeles. A study of how nursing students are socialized to cope with death was conducted as part of a larger study supported by Public Health Service Grant Nu00047 from the Division of Nursing, Bureau of State Services-Community Health, at the University of California, San Francisco. The social meanings of diabetes mellitus in adolescence was supported by a Special Nurse Fellowship (5F4-NU-10, 227-02) awarded by the Division of Nursing, National Institutes of Health.

REFERENCES

1. Ball, D. W. Toward a Sociology of Telephones and Telephoners. In M. Truzzi (Ed.), *Sociology and Everyday Life.* Englewood Cliffs, N. J.: Prentice-Hall, 1968, pp. 59–75.
2. Becker, H. S., and Geer, B. The Analysis of Qualitative Field Data. In R. N. Adams and J. J. Preiss (Eds.), *Human Organization Research.* Homewood, Ill.: Dorsey Press, 1960, pp. 279–289.
3. Bell, N., Trieschman, A., and Vogel, A. A sociocultural analysis of the resistances of working class fathers. *American Journal of Orthopsychiatry* 31:395–397, 1961.

4. Benedict, R. *Patterns of Culture.* Boston: Houghton Mifflin, 1934.
5. Benoliel, J. Q. The Developing Diabetic Identity: A Study of Family Influence. In M. V. Batey (Ed.), *Communicating Nursing Research: Methodological Issues.* Boulder, Colo.: WICHE, 1970, pp. 14–32.
6. Berelson, B. *Content Analysis in Communication Research.* Glencoe, Ill.: Free Press, 1952.
7. Blumer, H. *Symbolic Interactionism: Perspective and Method.* Englewood Cliffs, N. J.: Prentice-Hall, 1969.
8. Bregg, E. A., Leddy, M. C., and Mackenzie, L. G. "A Study on the Nurses' Concept of Death." (Ed.D. dissertation, Teachers College, Columbia University, 1953).
9. Bruyn, S. The methodology of participant observation. *Human Organization* 22:229–233, 1963.
10. Byerly, E. L. The nurse researcher as participant-observer in a nursing setting. *Nursing Research* 18:230–236, 1969.
11. Cicourel, A. V. *Method and Measurement in Sociology.* New York: Free Press, 1964, pp. 100–104.
12. Dean, J. P., and Whyte, W. F. How do you know if the informant is telling the truth? *Human Organization* 17:34–38, 1958.
13. Dickinson, A. R. "Nurses' Perceptions of Their Care of Patients Dying with Cancer." (Ed.D. dissertation, Teachers College, Columbia University, 1966).
14. Ellis, R. The nurse as investigator and member of the research team. *Annals of the New York Academy of Science* 169:435–441, 1970.
15. Erikson, K. T. A comment on disguised observations in sociology. *Social Problems* 14:366–381, 1967.
16. Feifel, H. Attitudes of Mentally Ill Patients Toward Death. In R. Fulton (Ed.), *Death and Identity.* New York: Wiley, 1965, pp. 131–142.
17. Folta, J. R. The perception of death. *Nursing Research* 14:232–235, 1965.
18. Fox, R. C. *Experiment Perilous.* Glencoe, Ill.: Free Press, 1959.
19. Fox, R. C. An American Sociologist in the Land of Belgian Medical Research. In P. E. Hammond (Ed.), *Sociologists At Work.* New York: Basic Books, 1964, pp. 345–391.
20. Garfinkel, H. *Studies in Ethnomethodology.* Englewood Cliffs, N. J.: Prentice-Hall, 1967, pp. 76–103.
21. Geer, G. First Days in the Field. In P. E. Hammond (Ed.), *Sociologists At Work.* New York: Basic Books, 1964, pp. 322–344.
22. Glaser, B. G. The constant comparative method of qualitative analysis. *Social Problems* 12:436–445, 1965.
23. Glaser, B. G., and Strauss, A. L. *Awareness of Dying.* Chicago: Aldine, 1965.
24. Glaser, B. G., and Strauss, A. L. *The Discovery of Grounded Theory: Strategies for Qualitative Research.* Chicago: Aldine, 1967, pp. 45–77.
25. Glaser, B. G., and Strauss, A. L. *Time for Dying.* Chicago: Aldine, 1968.
26. Glass, B. The ethical basis of science. *Science* 150:1254–1261, 1965.
27. Gunter, L. M. Research techniques applied to nursing. *Nursing Research* 13:231–232, 1964.

28. Hershey, N. Negligence. *American Journal of Nursing* 62:98–99, 1962.
29. Hershey, N. Nurses' medical practice problems, II. *American Journal of Nursing* 62:75–77, 1962.
30. Hooper, T., and Spilka, B. Some meanings and correlates of future time and death among college students. *Omega* 1:49–56, 1970.
31. Hyman, H. H., et al. *Interviewing in Social Research.* Chicago: University of Chicago Press, 1954.
32. Janes, R. W. A note on phases of the community role of the participant-observer. *American Sociological Review* 26:446–450, 1961.
33. Kahn, R., and Mann, F. Developing research partnerships. *Journal of Social Issues* 8:4–10, 1952.
34. McCall, G. J., and Simmons, J. L. *Issues in Participant Observation.* Reading, Mass.: Addison-Wesley, 1969, pp. 3–5, 128–141.
35. Mead, M. Research with human beings: A model derived from anthropological field practice. *Daedalus* 98:361–386, 1969.
36. Pearsall, M. Participant observation as role and method in behavioral research. *Nursing Research* 14:40–42, 1965.
37. Quint, J. C. An exploratory investigation of the process of adjustment following radical mastectomy. Application for Research Grant, University of California, Los Angeles, 1961.
38. Quint, J. C. Delineation of qualitative aspects of nursing care. *Nursing Research* 11:204–206, 1962.
39. Quint, J. C. The impact of mastectomy. *American Journal of Nursing* 63:88–91, 1963.
40. Quint, J. C. The First Year after Mastectomy: The Patients and the Nurse-Researchers. In *Designs for Nurse-Patient Interaction, Convention Clinical Sessions,* vol. 9. New York: American Nurses' Association, 1964, pp. 5–12.
41. Quint, J. C. Mastectomy – symbol of cure or warning sign? *GP* 29:119–124, 1964.
42. Quint, J. C. Institutionalized practices of information control. *Psychiatry* 28:119–132, 1965.
43. Quint, J. C. *The Nurse and the Dying Patient.* New York: Macmillan, 1967.
44. Quint, J. C. Research – how will nursing define it? The case for theories generated from empirical data. *Nursing Research* 16:109–114, 1967.
45. Quint, J. C. Some Thoughts on a Theory of Chronicity. In C. M. Norris (Ed.), *Proceedings, First Nursing Theory Conference.* University of Kansas Medical Center, Department of Nursing Education, 1969, pp. 58–67.
46. Quint, J. C. *Becoming Diabetic: A Study of Emerging Identity.* D. N. Sc. dissertation, University of California, San Francisco, 1969.
47. Rainwater, L., and Pittman, D. J. Ethical problems in studying a politically sensitive and deviant community. *Social Problems* 14:357–366, 1967.
48. Richardson, S. A., Dohrenwend, B. S., and Klein, D. *Interviewing: Its Forms and Functions.* New York: Basic Books, 1965, pp. 45–55 and 96–100.
49. Robinson, W. S. The logical structure of analytic induction. *American Sociological Review* 16:812–818, 1951.

50. Rosenthal, R. *Experimental Effects in Behavioral Research.* New York: Appleton-Century-Crofts, 1966.
51. Savard, R. J. Serving Investigator, Patient, and Community in Research Studies. *Annals of the New York Academy of Science* 169:429–434, 1970.
52. Schutz, A. Symbol, Reality, and Society. In L. Bryson et al., (Eds.), *Symbols and Society.* New York: Harper & Bros., 1955, pp. 150–156.
53. Schwartz, M. S., and Schwartz, C. G. Problems in participant observation. *The American Journal of Sociology* 60:343–353, 1955.
54. Smith, H. C. *Care of the Dying Patient: A Comparison of Instructional Plans.* Ed.D. dissertation, Indiana University, 1965.
55. Smith, M. B. Conflicting values affecting behavioral research with children. *Children* 14:53–58, 1967.
56. Strauss, A. L., et al. *Psychiatric Ideologies and Institutions.* New York: Free Press, 1964.
57. Sudnow, D. *Passing On – The Social Organization of Dying.* Englewood Cliffs, N. J.: Prentice-Hall, 1967.
58. Vidich, A. J. Participant observation and the collection and interpretation of data. *American Journal of Sociology* 60:354–360, 1955.
59. Waechter, E. H. *Death Anxiety in Children with Fatal Illness.* Ph.D. dissertation, Stanford University, 1968.
60. Wax, R. H. Reciprocity in Fieldwork. In R. N. Adams and J. J. Preiss (Eds.), *Human Organization in Research.* Homewood, Ill.: Dorsey, 1960, pp. 90–98.
61. Wolfensberger, W. Ethical issues in research with human subjects. *Science* 155:47–51, 1967.
62. Zelditch, M. Some methodological problems of field studies. *American Journal of Sociology* 67:566–576, 1962.

Index